The Transthoracic Examination

Bernard E. Bulwer, MD, MSc, FASE

Program Director, Diagnostic Medical Sonography-Echocardiography
Associate Professor
School of Medical Imaging and Therapeutics
MCPHS University
Boston, Massachusetts, USA

Noninvasive Cardiovascular Research
Brigham and Women's Hospital
Boston, Massachusetts, USA

José M. Rivero, MD

Chief Cardiac Sonographer
Cardiovascular Division
Brigham and Women's Hospital
Boston, Massachusetts, USA

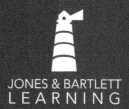

JONES & BARTLETT
LEARNING

World Headquarters
Jones & Bartlett Learning
5 Wall Street
Burlington, MA 01803
978-443-5000
info@jblearning.com
www.jblearning.com

Jones & Bartlett Learning books and products are available through most bookstores and online book-sellers. To contact Jones & Bartlett Learning directly, call 800-832-0034, fax 978-443-8000, or visit our website, www.jblearning.com.

Substantial discounts on bulk quantities of Jones & Bartlett Learning publications are available to corporations, professional associations, and other qualified organizations. For details and specific discount information, contact the special sales department at Jones & Bartlett Learning via the above contact information or send an email to specialsales@jblearning.com.

Some images in this book feature models. These models do not necessarily endorse, represent, or participate in the activities represented in the images.

The authors, editor, and publisher have made every effort to provide accurate information. However, they are not responsible for errors, omissions, or for any outcomes related to the use of the contents of this book and take no responsibility for the use of the products and procedures described. Treatments and side effects described in this book may not be applicable to all people; likewise, some people may require a dose or experience a side effect that is not described herein. Drugs and medical devices are discussed that may have limited availability controlled by the Food and Drug Administration (FDA) for use only in a research study or clinical trial. Research, clinical practice, and government regulations often change the accepted standard in this field. When consideration is being given to use of any drug in the clinical setting, the health care provider or reader is responsible for determining FDA status of the drug, reading the package insert, and reviewing prescribing information for the most up-to-date recommendations on dose, precautions, and contraindications, and determining the appropriate usage for the product. This is especially important in the case of drugs that are new or seldom used.

Production Credits

Publisher: Christopher Davis
Senior Acquisitions Editor: Alison Hankey
Special Projects Editor: Kathy Richardson
Editorial Assistant: Jessica Acox
Editorial Assistant: Sara Cameron
Senior Production Editor: Tracey Chapman
Senior Marketing Manager: Barb Bartoszek
V.P., Manufacturing and Inventory Control: Therese Connell
Composition: DSCS, LLC
Cover Design: Kristin E. Parker
Printing and Binding: Courier Digital Solutions
Cover Printing: Courier Digital Solutions

Library of Congress Cataloging-in-Publication Data
Bulwer, Bernard E.
    Echocardiography pocket guide : the transthoracic examination / Bernard E. Bulwer, José M. Rivero.
    p. ; cm.
    Includes bibliographical references and index.
    ISBN-13: 978-0-7637-7935-1 (pbk.)
    ISBN-10: 0-7637-7935-0 (pbk.)
    1. Echocardiography—Handbooks, manuals, etc.   I. Rivero, José M.   II. Title.
    [DNLM: 1. Echocardiography—Handbooks. WG 39 B941e 2009]
    RC683.5.U5B85 2009
    616.1'207543—dc22
                                                                    2009030410

6048

Printed in the United States of America
16 15 14 13 12   10 9 8 7 6 5 4 3 2

To the Awesome Giver of sight,
Who, when I was blind, made me see,
and when bound, set me free.

To: Scott and José for opening the doors to echocardiography; and Noor, Soon-il, Nino, Ya Ching, Mama, and my entire family, Ernest & Bunny Staine, John & Martha Woods, without whom this work would have remained but a dream, not reality.

B.E. Bulwer

CONTENTS OVERVIEW

PREFACE

A new impetus has emerged for a realistic step-by-step presentation of the transthoracic echocardiography examination. Wider availability, increased portability, and expanding applications have issued a new mandate for practical teaching aids for both the cardiologist and noncardiologist.

Echocardiography, or cardiac ultrasonography, has an established role in the diagnosis and management of patients with suspected and established heart disease. Miniaturization of this technology has given new meaning to the word "stethos-scope"—the ability to visualize cardiac structure and function, a feat far more clinically useful than the traditional auscultation of heart sounds. The arrival of such handheld and pocket-sized devices means that medical students, residents, fellows, and noncardiologists need the basic skills to perform and interpret at least a focused echocardiography examination. Such skills should lead to a deeper understanding of cardiac structure and function at the patient's bedside— an approach espoused by the American Society of Echocardiography (in competent hands). This can translate into improved point-of-care diagnosis, less delays to diagnosis, optimal referrals, and reduced costs.

Echocardiography is the sonographer's scalpel—a tool that greatly enhances our understanding of in vivo cardiac anatomy, physiology, and hemodynamics. As such, it can greatly complement medical education and allied health training.

With these goals in mind, *Echocardiography Pocket Guide: The Transthoracic Examination* presents a highly illustrated step-by-step introduction to the basics of the transthoracic examination. The typical sonographer scans the heart using his or her right hand while seated on the patient's right. Such views are shown throughout to demonstrate the examination. Views from the patient's left side are also presented, as many sonographers prefer scanning from this perspective. Views using the standard anatomical position, with the patient erect and facing the examiner, are included to maintain harmony with traditional anatomy education and other cardiac imaging techniques, such as computerized tomography (CT) and magnetic resonance imaging (MRI).

This guide's primary focus is the normal examination. However, it makes frequent references to salient pathologic findings that can be seen, and should be sought, on each view as the examination proceeds. In this pursuit, tabular summaries and panoramic illustrations of normal and abnormal findings of cardiac structure and function follow the presentation of each view. This reflects the systematic thought process that is executed by expert sonographers as the examination proceeds. Echocardiographic findings typically require confirmation using multiple views, and this three-dimensional perspective is emphasized. The major focus is the adult examination, but additional image projections that are used in the pediatric examination for evaluating congenital heart disease are sprinkled throughout. A Reference Guide of normal values for the quantification of cardiac chamber dimensions appears at the end of this volume.

We hope this guide fulfills its design.

—BEB and JMR

ACKNOWLEDGMENTS

To the wonderful cardiac sonographers of the Cardiovascular Division, Brigham and Women's Hospital. Special thanks to Faranak Farrohi, Kurt Jacobsen, and Khadija Ouannas.

To Professor Charles and Christiana Malgwi.

To all who encouraged us along the way to make this work a reality, in ways spoken and unspoken, to you we are indebted.

Singular thanks go to Mr. Leighton Brady, cardiac sonographer at the Brigham and Women's Hospital, for modeling his superb physique to demonstrate the normal echocardiographic examination.

FOREWORD

Echocardiography is a manual skill. Unlike other imaging techniques, where a patient is positioned and a technician may press a series of buttons, echocardiography requires that a skilled operator apply a transducer manually to a patient's thorax. Moreover, as echocardiography is not a tomographic technique, the images obtained are neither uniform nor guaranteed to be of a certain quality or even spatial location. Hence, the quality of the images obtained is directly dependent on that operator's skill and experience; the success of the examination begins and ends at the hands of the person holding the transducer.

Echocardiography Pocket Guide: The Transthoracic Examination by Bernard Bulwer and José Rivero, provides an introduction to cardiac imaging with echocardiography for anyone interested in learning this skill. It will appeal to sonographers in training and beyond. It will appeal to cardiology fellows, emergency physicians, and any physician or health professional interested in learning echocardiography from a hands-on perspective.

In addition to providing an expert introduction to the process of performing an echocardiographic examination, this book is expertly illustrated and will guide users through the first steps of interpreting echocardiographic images. A good sonographer needs to know what to look for, and how to look for it. While a solid understanding of the kinds of pathology that are typically seen are essential in an echocardiographers training, the most important thing an echocardiographer can learn is to recognize *normal*, as only then can he or she appreciate and understand deviations from normality.

As echocardiography transitions from a technology dominated by subspecialists to one that likely will be embraced by a growing number of practitioners, there will be a growing need for very practical instruction in this art, which has generally been taught by apprenticeship. This shift will likely be driven by the advent of smaller, more efficient and cheaper hand-held and portable echocardiographic devices that are beginning to transform cardiac imaging. This handbook has a central role in this transition, and will provide a wide range of clinicians with a foundation for the practice of the skills necessary for diagnosing patients using echocardiography.

Scott D. Solomon, MD
Professor of Medicine
Harvard Medical School
Director, Noninvasive Cardiology
Brigham and Women's Hospital
Deputy Editor, *Circulation*
Boston, MA

Echocardiography Basics

PART 1

CHAPTER 1

Introduction

ECHOCARDIOGRAPHY: DEFINITION

Echocardiography, or *cardiac ultrasonography,* uses ultrasound echoes reflected from the heart to generate images of cardiac structure and function Figure 1.1 .

In two-dimensional (2D) or cross-sectional echocardiography, the transducer scans through the anatomical scan plane. The reflected ultrasound echoes are processed and displayed in real time as a pie-shaped scan sector. Doppler echocardiography displays blood flow velocities as a color flow map or as a spectrum of velocities during the cardiac cycle Figure 1.1 . Modern echocardiography instruments

Figure 1.1

Basic overview of echocardiography—cardiac ultrasound imaging. Ultrasound is high-frequency inaudible sound, with frequencies greater than 20 kHz (20 × 10^3 cycles per second). To create the ultrasound image, ultrasound must be transmitted, reflected, processed, and displayed.

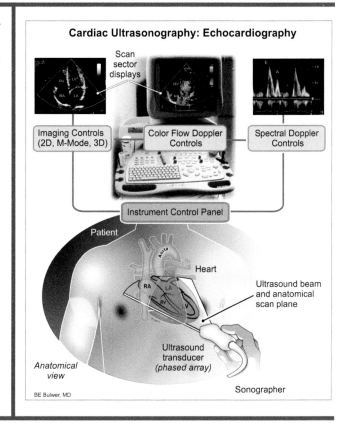

Cardiac Ultrasonography: Echocardiography

Scan sector displays

Imaging Controls (2D, M-Mode, 3D)

Color Flow Doppler Controls

Spectral Doppler Controls

Instrument Control Panel

Patient

Aorta

Heart

RA LA

RV

Ultrasound beam and anatomical scan plane

Ultrasound transducer (phased array)

Anatomical view

Sonographer

BE Bulwer, MD

use phased array transducer technology. Phased array transducers have two important design features that are suited for echocardiography:

1. They occupy a small "footprint," which is ideal for scanning through the narrow intercostal spaces (as the ribs greatly attenuate the ultrasound beam)
2. Their electronic beam steering feature facilitates scanning through a comparatively wide anatomical scan plane, despite their small footprint

BASIC TYPES OF ECHOCARDIOGRAPHY

Two fundamental properties of ultrasound are used to derive information about cardiac structure and function.

Anatomical or B-mode echocardiography relies primarily on the relative strengths or amplitudes (wave height above baseline) of the reflected ultrasound echoes to determine their "echoreflectivity," or degree of brightness, on the image display.

Doppler echocardiography, in contrast, analyzes the change or shift in frequency (of the received echoes compared to the transmitted echoes) to determine the velocities of blood flow and myocardial tissue motion Table 1.1 .

The use of ultrasound contrast agents (contrast echocardiography) can enhance B-mode and Doppler echocardiography. Speckle tracking echocardiography is an analytical technique that tracks movement of B-mode structures throughout the cardiac cycle to provide information about cardiac motion, velocity, and deformation.

Table 1.1 B-MODE ECHOCARDIOGRAPHY AND DOPPLER ECHOCARDIOGRAPHY COMPARED

	B-mode echocardiography (M-mode, 2D, 3D)	Doppler echocardiography	Tissue Doppler echocardiography
Clinical utility	Cardiac structure	Cardiac function	Cardiac function
Discipline	Anatomy	Physiology and hemodynamics	Myocardial mechanics
Target tissues/ region of interest	Myocardium, pericardium, endocardium, heart valves, great vessels	Blood cells (blood flow)	Myocardium (tissue motion)
Parameters measured	Morphology (relative size, shape)	Direction, velocity, flow pattern	Direction, velocity, deformation
Optimal ultrasound beam alignment	Perpendicular	Parallel	Parallel

2D: two-dimensional; 3D: three-dimensional; B-mode: brightness mode; M-mode: motion-mode (one-dimensional motion-mode over time).

CLINICAL VALUE OF ECHOCARDIOGRAPHY

Echocardiography is the most widely used cardiac imaging technique. It has a clinically proven role in the diagnosis and management of patients with suspected or established cardiovascular disease Table 1.2 .

Table 1.2 THE CLINICAL APPLICATIONS OF ECHOCARDIOGRAPHY

Symptoms or presentation	Clinical signs	Medical conditions	Screening
Suspected cardiac etiology in patients with: • Dyspnea • Chest pain • Lightheadedness • TIA • Cerebrovascular events • Syncope • Cyanosis • Hypotension • Hemodynamic instability • Respiratory failure	Cardiac murmurs: systolic, diastolic, continuous, thrills, mid-systolic click	Heart failure (CHF)	Left ventricular hypertrophy (LVH) (hypertension)
		Coronary artery disease (CAD)	Abdominal aortic aneurysm
	Cardiomegaly or enlarged cardiac silhouette on CXR	Cardiomyopathies	LVH in familial cardiomyopathies, e.g., hypertrophic cardiomyopathy
	Hypertension	Arrhythmias: AF, SVT, VT; pacing device evaluation	Athletes with family history of sudden cardiac death
	Hypotension	Stroke	Left atrial enlargement
	Arrhythmias, esp. if sustained, e.g., AF, SVT, VT	Valvular heart disease	Left ventricular (LV) dysfunction
Acute coronary syndromes (ACS)	Low voltage on ECG	Infective endocarditis	Right ventricular (RV) dysfunction
Hypertension		Pericardial disease	Valvular heart disease
Cardiac arrest		Pulmonary embolism	
Heart failure (CHF)		Pulmonary hypertension	Pericardial effusion
Multiple trauma		Diseases of the aorta	
		Hypertension	
		Diabetes	
		Family history of cardiomyopathies	
		Congenital heart disease	

AF: atrial fibrillation; TIA: transient ischemic attack; CXR: chest X-ray; ECG: electrocardiogram; SVT: supraventricular tachycardia; VT: ventricular tachycardia

ADVANTAGES OF ECHOCARDIOGRAPHY

Echocardiography is the most versatile cardiac imaging technique. It can provide a wide range of clinically useful information in a variety of settings, and at less cost, with more rapid results, as compared to other cardiac imaging techniques Table 1.3 .

Highly portable battery-powered instruments, known as hand-carried ultrasound (HCU), can be used outside the hospital setting in locations such as community clinics, resource-poor environments, ambulances, and aircraft (even spacecraft). Up-and-coming pocket-sized devices have been dubbed as the "ultrasound stethoscopes" of the future.

Table 1.3 ADVANTAGE OF ECHOCARDIOGRAPHY COMPARED TO OTHER CARDIAC IMAGING TECHNIQUES

Advantages	
Excellent diagnostic utility	Established role in the diagnosis, management, risk stratification, and prognosis in patients with suspected or established cardiovascular disease; Safety established in adults, pregnancy, and children
Safe, highly portable, and versatile	Inpatient and outpatient use; Highly portable and battery-powered forms can be used in community and remote settings; Transesophageal echocardiography is used in real time during cardiac surgery (without interrupting surgical procedures); Ultrasound stethoscope and futuristic "cell phone" of cardiac imaging concept
Immediate results	Highly portable; New ultraportable hand-carried and pocket-sized instruments slated to become the future ultrasound "stethoscope"
Less expensive and wider availability	Compared to cardiac computerized tomography (CT), cardiac magnetic resonance imaging (C-MRI), and nuclear cardiology imaging; Safe in pregnancy and childhood
No radiation	Compared to cardiac CT and nuclear cardiology imaging
Minimal patient discomfort	No need for breath-holding as with C-MRI; Rapid image acquisition times: New 3D echocardiography imaging can be obtained during one heart beat—drastically reducing image acquisition times; Reduced need for scanning expertise: New 3D echocardiography instruments require less scanning expertise

SKILLS AND COMPETENCY: THE REQUISITES

Standards for performance and interpretation of echocardiographic studies have been established and endorsed by expert bodies like the American Society of Echocardiography (ASE), the American College of Cardiology (ACC), the American Heart Association, and their European and British counterparts Table 1.4 .

Table 1.4 REQUISITE SKILLS AND COMPETENCY
IN ECHOCARDIOGRAPHY

Basic Cognitive Skills Required for Competence in Echocardiography *(ACC/AHA/ASE, 2003)*
- Knowledge of physical principles of echocardiographic image formation and blood flow velocity measurements.
- Knowledge of instrument settings required to obtain an optimal image.
- Knowledge of normal cardiac anatomy.
- Knowledge of pathologic changes in cardiac anatomy due to acquired and CHD.
- Knowledge of fluid dynamics of normal blood flow.
- Knowledge of pathological changes in blood flow due to acquired heart disease and CHD.

CHD: congenital heart disease

Cognitive Skills Required for Competence in Adult Transthoracic Echocardiography *(ACC/AHA/ASE, 2003)*
- Basic knowledge outlined above.
- Knowledge of appropriate indications for echocardiography.
- Knowledge of the differential diagnostic problem in each case and the echocardiographic techniques required to investigate these possibilities.
- Knowledge of appropriate transducer manipulation.
- Knowledge of cardiac auscultation and electrocardiography for correlation with results of the echocardiogram.
- Ability to distinguish an adequate from an inadequate echocardiographic examination.
- Knowledge of appropriate semi-quantitative and quantitative measurement techniques and ability to distinguish adequate from inadequate quantitation.
- Ability to communicate results of the examination to the patient, medical record, and other physicians.
- Knowledge of alternatives to echocardiography.

CHAPTER 2

Echocardiographic Anatomy, Windows, and Imaging Planes

IN THE DESCRIPTION OF THE HUMAN BODY, all terms are used in relation to the anatomic position, which by convention is defined as one in which the body is viewed in its erect position, the head, eyes, and toes directed anteriorly, the arms by the side and supinated—the descriptions of cardiac anatomy are often unique in their disregard for this cardinal principle.

Wallace A. McAlpine, MD, FRCS
Heart and Coronary Arteries (1975)

ANATOMICAL VERSUS ECHOCARDIOGRAPHIC IMAGING PLANES

Figure 2.1

The major axis of the heart, the long axis of the left ventricle (LV), is obliquely positioned and typically rotated ~60° away from the median plane in normal adults. This axis projects along a line extending from the right mid-clavicle to the palpable LV apical impulse *(upper left)*. This major cardiac axis serves as the anatomical reference for the standard echocardiographic imaging planes: long-axis (LAX), short-axis (SAX), and four-chamber (4C) planes *(bottom right)*.

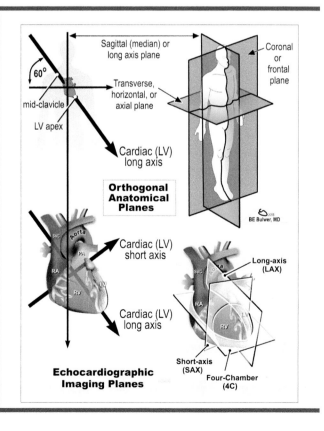

SURFACE ANATOMY OF THE HEART
Figure 2.2

Surface anatomy of the heart. *MCL: mid-clavicular line; LNL: left nipple line. See* Table 2.1 for accompanying labels.

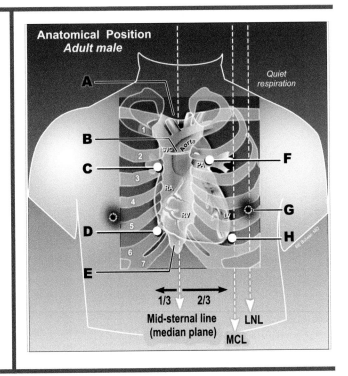

Table 2.1 SURFACE ANATOMY OF THE HEART

A	Suprasternal notch (SSN)	**E**	Xiphisternum (xiphoid process)
B	Manubrosternal angle (of Louis) - 2nd costal cartilage - Superior-inferior mediastinum border or transthoracic plane - Superior vena cava (SVC) begins - Arch of aorta begins and ends - Trachéal bifurcation - T4-T5 intervertebral disc	**F**	Left upper heart margin: inferior border of 2nd left costal cartilage
C	Right upper heart margin: superior border of 3rd chondrosternal junction	**G**	Left nipple (~4th ICS in males)
D	Right lower heart margin: 6th chondrosternal junction	**H**	Left ventricular (LV) apex: ~5th ICS - MCL

ICS: intercostal space; LNL: left nipple line; MCL: mid-clavicular line.

The heart, pericardium, and great vessels occupy the middle mediastinum—the portion of the chest cavity that lies in the midline between the two lungs and inferior to the palpable manubriosternal angle (Figures 2.2 and 2.3). The lungs enwrap the heart (and pericardium) laterally and over much of its anterolateral and posterolateral surfaces. Superiorly the great vessels—superior vena cava (SVC), ascending aorta, aortic arch and branches, and the main pulmonary artery (MPA) and bifurcation—enter and exit. Inferiorly, the heart sits on the diaphragm, through which passes the inferior vena cava (IVC) as it enters the floor of the right atrium. The heart's anterior or sternocostal surface is related to these structures: the sternum and the costal cartilages (ribs). Posteriorly, the heart's left atrium, which receives a pair of right and left pulmonary veins, lies immediately anterior to the esophagus.

Table 2.2 ANATOMICAL AND TOPOGRAPHICAL VARIANTS

Causes of variation in cardiac position and topography
1. Normal individual variation: e.g., long narrow vertical heart, more horizontal globular heart
2. Position of the body: erect, recumbent, lateral decubitus
3. Body habitus: including obesity and pregnancy
4. Phase of respiration and the cardiac cycle
5. Age: infants, children, elderly (heart of fetus and newborn more horizontal; apex swings downward in adulthood—heart more vertical
6. Diseases of the heart and pericardium, e.g., cardiomegaly, pericardial effusion, dextrocardia
7. Diseases of the chest wall: scoliosis, pectus excavatum
8. Diseases of the mediastinal structures
9. Lung disease: e.g., emphysema, pneumothorax
10. Post-chest surgery

WINDOWS, IMAGING PLANES, AND STANDARD VIEWS
Figure 2.3

In two-dimensional echocardiography, each cross-sectional view of the heart is described using three standard components: 1. The position or window from which the heart is viewed; 2. The major cardiac anatomical reference plane used to "slice" the heart—long-axis (LAX), short-axis (SAX), and four-chamber (4C); and 3. The particular region of interest or cardiac structures recorded.

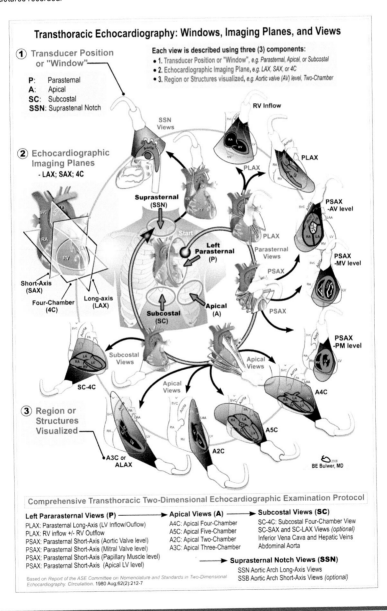

Transthoracic Echocardiography: Windows, Imaging Planes, and Views

(1) Transducer Position or "Window"

Each view is described using three (3) components:
- 1. Transducer Position or "Window", e.g. Parasternal, Apical, or Subcostal
- 2. Echocardiographic Imaging Plane, e.g. LAX, SAX, or 4C
- 3. Region or Structures visualized, e.g. Aortic valve (AV) level, Two-Chamber

P: Parasternal
A: Apical
SC: Subcostal
SSN: Suprasternal Notch

(2) Echocardiographic Imaging Planes
- LAX; SAX; 4C

Short-Axis (SAX)
Four-Chamber (4C)
Long-axis (LAX)

Suprasternal (SSN)
Left Parasternal (P)
Subcostal (SC)
Apical (A)

SSN Views
RV Inflow
PLAX
PLAX
PSAX -AV level
PSAX -MV level
PSAX
PSAX -PM level
Parasternal Views
Subcostal Views
SC-4C
Apical Views
Apical Views
A4C
A5C
A2C
A3C or ALAX

(3) Region or Structures Visualized

BE Bulwer, MD

Comprehensive Transthoracic Two-Dimensional Echocardiographic Examination Protocol

Left Pararasternal Views (P)
PLAX: Parasternal Long-Axis (LV Inflow/Outflow)
PLAX: RV inflow +/- RV Outflow
PSAX: Parasternal Short-Axis (Aortic Valve level)
PSAX: Parasternal Short-Axis (Mitral Valve level)
PSAX: Parasternal Short-Axis (Papillary Muscle level)
PSAX: Parasternal Short-Axis (Apical LV level)

Apical Views (A)
A4C: Apical Four-Chamber
A5C: Apical Five-Chamber
A2C: Apical Two-Chamber
A3C: Apical Three-Chamber

Subcostal Views (SC)
SC-4C: Subcostal Four-Chamber View
SC-SAX and SC-LAX Views *(optional)*
Inferior Vena Cava and Hepatic Veins
Abdominal Aorta

Suprasternal Notch Views (SSN)
SSN Aortic Arch Long-Axis Views
SSB Aortic Arch Short-Axis Views *(optional)*

Based on Report of the ASE Committee on Nomenclature and Standards in Two-Dimensional Echocardiography. Circulation. 1980 Aug;62(2):212-7

THE STANDARD TRANSDUCER POSITIONS (WINDOWS)

Echocardiographic images are acquired by placing the transducer (with acoustic coupling gel) at specific locations on the chest or abdominal wall Figures 2.3, 2.4, 2.10–2.13a and 2.13b : (i) Left parasternal (P) position or window, (ii) Left apical (A) position or window, (iii) Subcostal (SC), and (iv) Suprasternal (SSN) position or window.

Individual patient characteristics and the clinical indications for the examination will dictate whether all windows are used, or if additional nonstandard windows should be exploited. For example, in adults with congenital heart disease or following chest wall surgery, use whatever windows are available that provide optimal visualization of the desired views. The right parasternal window (R-PLAX) mirrors that of the left. It can provide optimal assessment of peak blood flow velocities in patients with aortic stenosis because of its more parallel alignment with left ventricular and aortic outflow tracts (see R-PLAX window, Figures 10.1 and 10.2).

A comprehensive transthoracic echocardiographic examination requires assessment using multiple views or perspectives. Composite views deliver a three-dimensional (3D) perspective, and as a general rule, this is the requisite standard for accurate assessment of cardiac structure and function. However, the air-filled lungs and the bony chest wall are the greatest obstacles to the transmission of ultrasound beam. This imposes the need for "windows" to avoid the lungs and bony ribs, thereby optimizing visualization of cardiac structures Figure 2.3 .

Although these echocardiographic windows are a useful starting point, the final "decider" is to use those window(s) that provide optimal visualization of the cardiac structures of interest. Experienced cardiac sonographers rapidly scan the chest wall using broad transducer strokes to get a quick impression of which windows most readily yield the best views.

Figure 2.4

The standard echocardiographic windows or transducer positions. Because the bony chest wall and lungs act as major obstacles to ultrasound beam transmission, paths that minimize such interference serve as echocardiographic imaging "windows" to the heart. The limitations imposed by the bony chest wall do not apply to echocardiography in the fetus and the newborn infant.

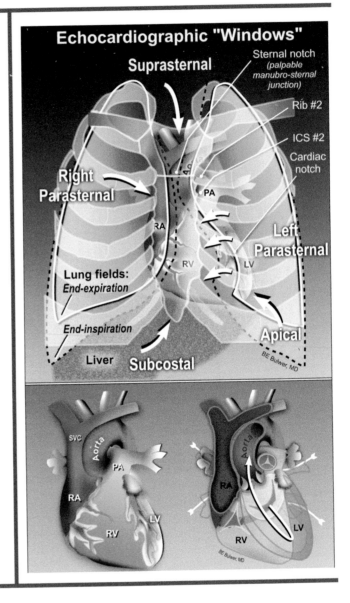

STANDARD ECHOCARDIOGRAPHIC IMAGING PLANES
Figure 2.5

Echocardiographic imaging planes. The anatomical reference for these planes is the long axis of the left ventricle (LV). There is an almost limitless number or family of anatomical planes that can be recorded as the transducer beam sweeps across the heart. For this reason, the reference standards used in echocardiography are the three primary orthogonal planes: LAX, SAX, and 4C. These transect the long- and short-axes of the heart.

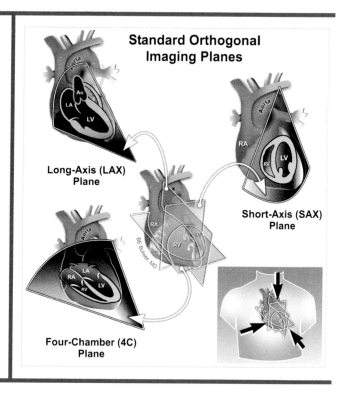

The long-axis plane extends from the LV apex to the aortic root (Ao), including the mitral and aortic valves. Surface markings of the long-axis plane approximate an imaginary line drawn from the right shoulder to the left loin (kidney). Long-axis planes of the left ventricle (LV) can be acquired from both the left parasternal and apical windows Figures 2.3, 2.5–2.7 .

Short-axis planes are obtained by transecting the heart perpendicular to the LV long axis, starting from the base of the heart (the plane of the atrioventricular junction), and "bread slicing" downward toward the apex. Surface markings of the primary short-axis plane approximate an imaginary line drawn from the mid-left clavicle to the right hip. Short-axis planes of the left ventricle can be viewed from both the left parasternal and subcostal windows Figures 2.3, 2.5–2.7 .

Four-chamber planes provide views of four cardiac chambers by transecting both the interventricular and interatrial septae in a plane perpendicular to the long and short axes. Surface markings of the four-chamber plane subtend across an imaginary line drawn from the LV apex to the right shoulder. Four-chamber planes of the left ventricle can be acquired from both the apical and subcostal windows Figures 2.3, 2.5–2.7 .

IMAGING PLANES AND CARDIAC ANATOMY

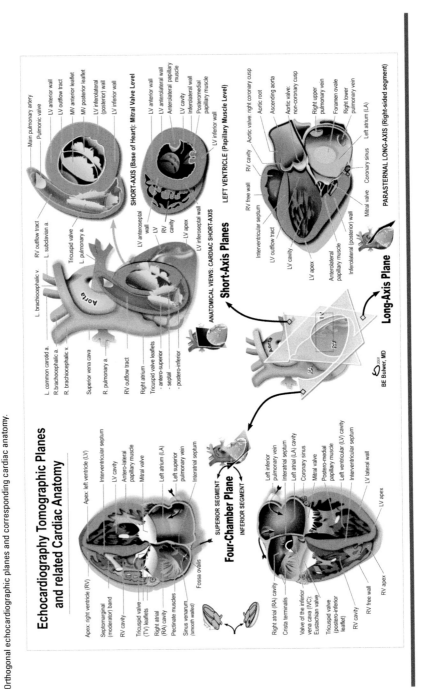

Figure 2.6

Orthogonal echocardiographic planes and corresponding cardiac anatomy.

THREE-DIMENSIONAL PERSPECTIVES
Figure 2.7

Three-dimensional (3D) views of the heart along the three standard echocardiographic planes: the four-chamber, short-axis, and long-axis planes.

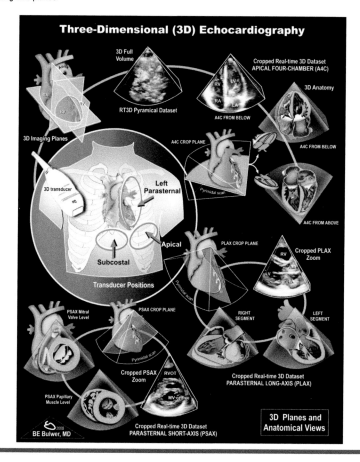

In three-dimensional (3D) echocardiography, full-volume pyramidal datasets can be acquired from the parasternal, apical, and subcostal windows. The acquired volumes can be cropped to yield cross-sectional views (with a 3D perspective) along the standard orthogonal echocardiographic imaging planes Figure 2.7 .

Current advantages of 3D over 2D echocardiography include: (i) more rapid image acquisition times, (ii) less operator dependence—less need for scanning expertise, and (iii) more accurate quantification of cardiac dimensions and volumes. However, because of the additional technical demands required to generate large 3D datasets using ultrasound, 3D images exhibit less detail (inferior spatial resolution), compared to 2D echocardiography.

ECHOCARDIOGRAPHIC IMAGING PLANES AND CORONARY ARTERY TERRITORIES

Ischemic heart disease and acute coronary syndromes are the leading cause of cardiac morbidity and mortality, and knowledge of the cardiac blood supply is a requisite for optimal assessment of echocardiographic findings. This is especially true for wall motion assessment. Ventricular walls that demonstrate abnormal movement and thickening, e.g., hypokinetic, akinetic, dyskinetic, aneurysmal, or thinned (scarred) walls, most commonly do so because of insults to the corresponding coronary artery supply. Therefore, regional wall motion abnormalities can support or negate the diagnosis in acute and chronic coronary syndromes.

Caveat: During the echocardiography examination, have a mental map of the coronary artery territory that corresponds to the various ventricular walls and segments Figures 2.8, 2.9 .

Figure 2.8

Coronary artery territories and the reference echocardiographic imaging planes. *LAA: left atrial appendage; LAD: left anterior descending coronary artery; LCx: left circumflex coronary artery; LMA: left main coronary artery; PDA: posterior descending (branch of the right coronary) artery; RCA: right coronary artery.*

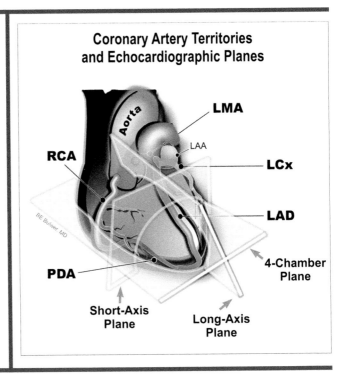

Coronary Artery Territories and Echocardiographic Planes

ECHOCARDIOGRAPHIC IMAGING PLANES, CORONARY ARTERY TERRITORIES, AND LEFT VENTRICULAR SEGMENTS (ASE)
Figure 2.9

Three-dimensional perspectives of left ventricular segmentation (polar or "bull's eye" plot), based on standards set by the American Society of Echocardiography (ASE). Although much variation and overlap exists in coronary artery supply, the most common pattern of coronary artery supply to the heart and left ventricular segments is shown.

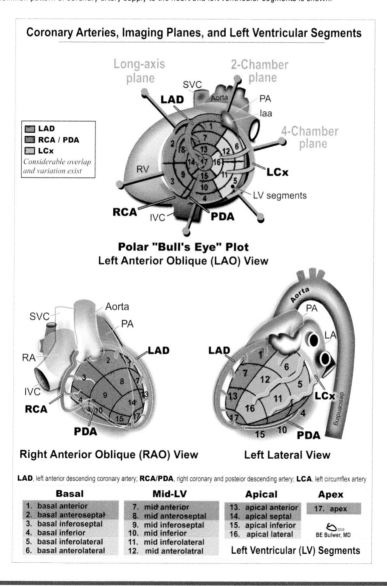

Coronary Arteries, Imaging Planes, and Left Ventricular Segments

Polar "Bull's Eye" Plot
Left Anterior Oblique (LAO) View

Right Anterior Oblique (RAO) View

Left Lateral View

LAD, left anterior descending coronary artery; **RCA/PDA**, right coronary and posteior descending artery; **LCA**, left circumflex artery

Basal	Mid-LV	Apical	Apex
1. basal anterior	7. mid anterior	13. apical anterior	17. apex
2. basal anteroseptal	8. mid anteroseptal	14. apical septal	
3. basal inferoseptal	9. mid inferoseptal	15. apical inferior	BE Bulwer, MD
4. basal inferior	10. mid inferior	16. apical lateral	
5. basal inferolateral	11. mid inferolateral		
6. basal anterolateral	12. mid anterolatral		

Left Ventricular (LV) Segments

PATIENT POSITIONING, WINDOWS, AND VIEWS

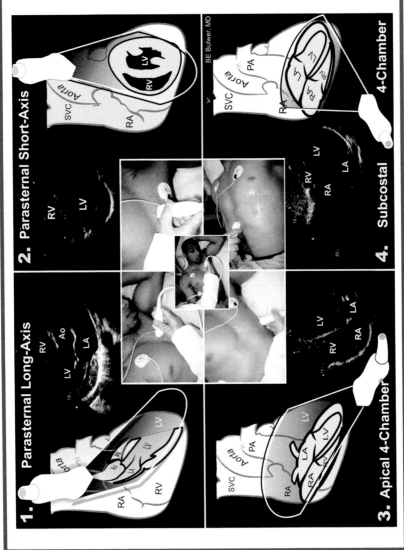

Figure 2.10

Optimal acquisition of echocardiographic views also requires optimal patient positioning. Plates 1 to 4 are a panoramic overview of patient positioning, transducer windows, and the corresponding echocardiographic view.

For most patients who can remain comfortable lying, the optimal patient position for the parasternal view is the left lateral decubitus position, as shown in Figures 2.10, 2.11, 2.12 . This is primarily because the left parasternal window—the area adjacent to the left sternal border that is created by the "cardiac notch" because of absence of a middle lobe of the left lung—is increased by gravity's pull on the lung away from the heart, and the heart's movement closer to the chest wall. For this reason, the apical views are best recorded when the patient is in the left lateral decubitus position. In contrast, the subcostal views are best obtained with the patient lying supine or semirecumbent and in end-expiration, which moves the heart closer to the transducer.

PATIENT POSITIONING, WINDOWS, AND ANATOMY
Figure 2.11

Surface anatomy of the standard echocardiogaphic windows with the patient in the left lateral decubitus position.

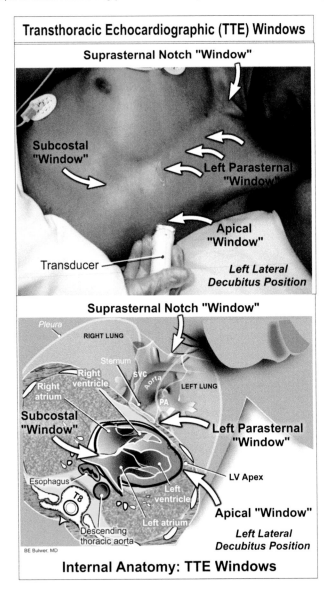

Figure 2.12

Corresponding internal anatomy with patient lying in the left lateral decubitus position. This position is generally best for obtaining the left parasternal and apical views.

Figure 2.13a

The standard transthoracic echocardiographic windows and relations with the major mediastinal organs (excluding lungs) and upper-abdominal anatomy, viewed from the patient's left side. Knowledge of these anatomical relationships is necessary, and it is the perspective seen when sonographers examine the heart from the patient's left side.

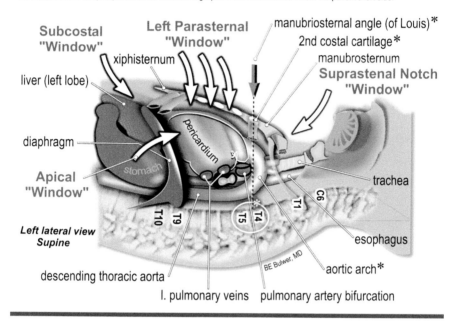

The structures highlighted in [Figure 2.13a] with the asterisk (*) serve as useful landmarks. The manubriosternal (sternal) angle corresponds to the intervertebral disc between the fourth (T4) and fifth (T5) thoracic vertebrae (see [Table 2.1] for other internal anatomical relationships at this level). The ribs are best counted using the palpable manubriosternal angle as the starting point. This corresponds to the second costal cartilage, below which lies the second intercostal space.

Note the relationship of the esophagus as it descends into the thorax [Figures 2.13a and 2.13b]. These relationships are important in transesophageal echocardiography. At the midesophageal level, the esophagus is intimately related to the left atrium—an important feature for orientation and interpretation of transesophageal echocardiography images.

Echocardiography is, in essence, functional cardiac anatomy and hemodynamics. In contrast to teaching methods based on traditional cardiac anatomical dissections or cadaver-based depictions of the heart, echocardiography provides real-time exhibition of *in vivo* cardiac structure and function.

Because echocardiography is safe, highly portable, and the most widely used cardiac imaging technique, it holds promise as a complementary tool in medical education. As echocardiography continues its natural evolution into smaller pocket-sized and hand-held devices, a prerequisite for its effective use is a sound knowledge of cardiac anatomy that resembles the live beating heart. Echocardiography, in this sense, is the ideal cardiac anatomy teaching tool.

Figure 2.13b

Mediastinal and upper-abdominal anatomy (left-sided view, erect) and their relationship to the transthoracic echocardiographic windows.

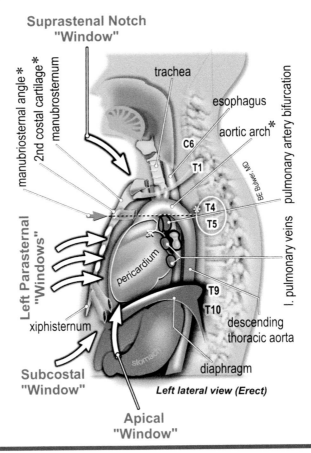

CHAPTER **3**

Instrumentation and Basic Principles of Echocardiography

OPTIMAL IMAGE ACQUISITION AND INSTRUMENT CONTROLS

Optimal acquisition, display, and interpretation of echocardiographic images requires a sound understanding of practical ultrasound physics, instrument control settings, individual patient characteristics, and their collective impact on the technical and diagnostic quality of echocardiographic data [Figure 3.1].

Figure 3.1

A requisite for optimal echoardiographic image acquisition and interpretation is the need to optimize the interplay between three key variables: the patient, the operator, and the instrument (see Figure 3.4 and Table 3.1).

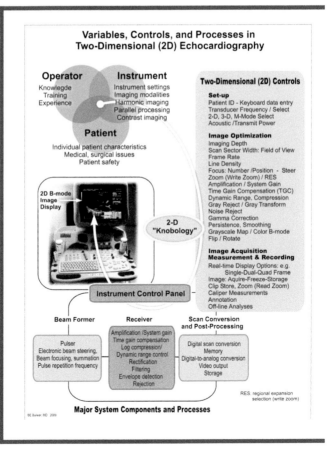

Variables, Controls, and Processes in Two-Dimensional (2D) Echocardiography

Operator
Knowlegde
Training
Experience

Instrument
Instrument settings
Imaging modalities
Harmonic imaging
Parallel processing
Contrast imaging

Patient
Individual patient characteristics
Medical, surgical issues
Patient safety

2D B-mode Image Display

2-D "Knobology"

Instrument Control Panel

Two-Dimensional (2D) Controls

Set-up
Patient ID - Keyboard data entry
Transducer Frequency / Select
2-D, 3-D, M-Mode Select
Acoustic /Transmit Power

Image Optimization
Imaging Depth
Scan Sector Width: Field of View
Frame Rate
Line Density
Focus: Number /Position - Steer
Zoom (Write Zoom) / RES
Amplification / System Gain
Time Gain Compensation (TGC)
Dynamic Range, Compression
Gray Reject / Gray Transform
Noise Reject
Gamma Correction
Persistence, Smoothing
Grayscale Map / Color B-mode
Flip / Rotate

Image Acquisition Measurement & Recording
Real-time Display Options: e.g.
Single-Dual-Quad Frame
Image: Aquire-Freeze-Storage
Clip Store, Zoom (Read Zoom)
Caliper Measurements
Annotation
Off-line Analyses

Beam Former
Pulser
Electronic beam steering,
Beam focusing, summation
Pulse repetition frequency

Receiver
Amplification /System gain
Time gain compensation
Log compression/
Dynamic range control
Rectification
Filtering
Envelope detection
Rejection

Scan Conversion and Post-Processing
Digital scan conversion
Memory
Digital-to-analog conversion
Video output
Storage

RES: regional expansion selection (write zoom)

Major System Components and Processes

BE Bulwer, MD 2009

Figure 3.2

Cardiac sonographer and echocardiography instrument during the examination. Knowledge of instrument controls or "knobology," akin to those of a car or airplane, is a prerequisite for optimal image acquisition and interpretation in echocardiography. Note the dim lighting used during the examination. Appropriate lighting is necessary to optimize image contrast, as excessive gain settings would be required when images are viewed using standard room lighting. This commonly occurs when echocardiography is performed in the operating theatre, where the intensity of the ambient lighting is high.

The instrument control panel or console has standard operational inputs via a standard keyboard and trackball in addition to ultrasound imaging and Doppler controls shown in Figures 3.3 and 3.4.

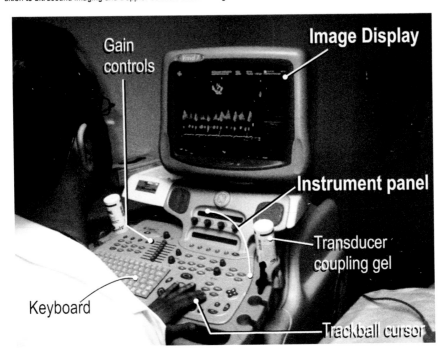

Figure 3.3

Top. Transducers and imaging and Doppler controls. Phased array transducers are the standard in echocardiography. They occupy a small "footprint" that facilitates scanning through the intercostal spaces (see Figures 3.6, 3.9, and 3.11). Switching between imaging modes, e.g., 2D (two-dimensional imaging), or M-mode (motion-mode over time or one-dimensional imaging), and Doppler modes, e.g., CW (continuous-wave Doppler) and PW (pulsed-wave Doppler), is easily executed by the switch of a button. *Bottom.* Modern phased array transducers are multifunctional and used for both anatomical imaging and Doppler studies *(left).* Nonimaging or Pedoff transducers are dedicated Doppler transducers.

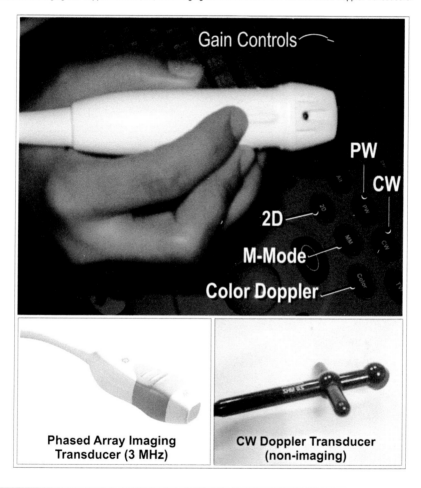

Phased Array Imaging Transducer (3 MHz)

CW Doppler Transducer (non-imaging)

A tradeoff exists when deciding which transducer to use. High-frequency transducers, e.g., 7.5 megahertz (MHz) or 5 MHz, can provide superior resolution (imaging detail), but are only appropriate for use in newborns and small infants, or for imaging more superficial cardiac structures like the cardiac apex. Low-frequency transducers, e.g., 2 to 3 MHz, penetrate more deeply and are suitable for the average adult examination, but they provide lower-resolution images.

MODERN INSTRUMENT CONTROL PANEL
Figure 3.4

Instrument panel on a modern cardiac ultrasound scanner. Knowledge of the major components, controls, and functions are key to optimal image acquisition and interpretation (see Table 3.1).

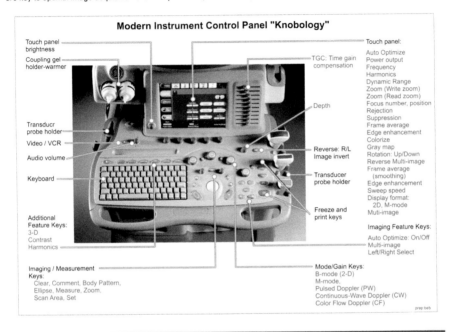

There are multiple imaging and Doppler controls used during the echocardiography examination. Optimal use of the technology requires familiarity with the instrument, as well as the principles underlying such instrument controls. One such control is time or depth gain compensation (TGC/DGC). The rationale for TGC controls is that image quality decays because of attenuation or loss of ultrasound strength with imaging depth. Making the appropriate adjustments compensates for such loss Figure 3.5 .

Figure 3.5

Composite schema showing the time-gain (or depth-gain) compensation principle. As ultrasound travels from the transducer to the imaged target, progressive attenuation or loss of strength or amplitude occurs *(upper left and central panel)*. To compensate those echoes that suffered more loss because of longer distance traveled——and to improve the attenuated image quality——the appropriate TGC is applied by adjusting the TGC sliding controls *(bottom panels)*.

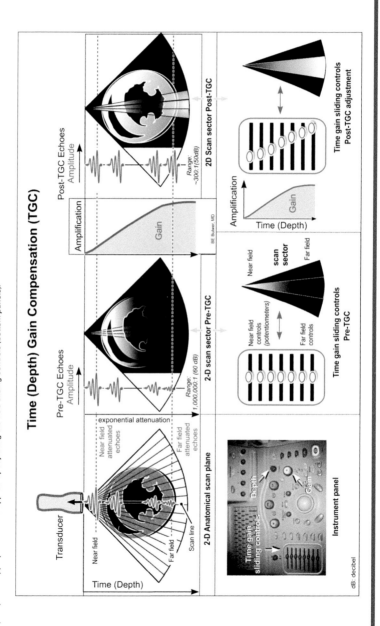

Time (Depth) Gain Compensation (TGC)

dB: decibel

SELECTED KNOBOLOGY AND INSTRUMENTATION BASICS

Table 3.1 SELECTED IMAGING GLOSSARY: CARDIAC ULTRASOUND INSTRUMENTATION "KNOBOLOGY"

2D	Two-dimensional echocardiography; commonly referred to as "B-mode"
3D	Three-dimensional echocardiography
Acoustic power	Transmit power; acoustic energy output of the ultrasound beam per unit time (in watts (W); control feature that adjusts the amount of energy delivered to the patient; use high-power default setting to optimize image quality (better signal-to-noise ratio); acoustic output indices: mechanical index (MI) and thermal index (TI) typically displayed on image frame
Amplitude	Ultrasound wave height above baseline; a basic physical characteristic of sound waves that is used in processing B-mode or gray scale images; ultrasound beam energy, intensity, and power are closely related
Annotation keys	Function keys to enter labels or measurements on the B-mode image display
Archiving	Transferring echo images to storage media, e.g., CDs, DVDs, flash drives
Artifact	Imaging artifact; false representations of the imaged tissue; can result from operator, instrument settings, and patient factors
B-color	*See* color B-mode
B-mode	Brightness modulation of amplitudes of the received echo signals using gray scale; display formats include M-mode, 2D, and 3D options
Calipers	Function tools for measurements, typically activated by pointing device
Cine loop/playback	For review of recently acquired images within system memory before applying freeze or save functions
Coded excitation	Technique for improving far field image resolution and penetration
Color B-mode	B-mode contrast-enhancing technique using various color options
Colorize	*See* color B-mode
Compression	Postprocessing setting which, in conjunction with log compression (dynamic range control that is a preprocessing function), improves or softens the appearance of B-mode images
Depth	Distance from the transducer; adjust as needed to visualize specified region of interest; depth scale visible on scan sector; frame rate decreased with greater imaging depth because of finite speed of ultrasound
Depth gain	Depth gain compensation (DGC); *See* Time gain compensation (TGC)
Dynamic range/log compression	Range of echo intensities ranging from threshold (smallest) to saturation (largest) that can be displayed on the B-mode ultrasound image; increasing the dynamic range increases the number of gray shades (improved contrast resolution); decreasing the dynamic range decreases number of gray shades (decreased contrast resolution—image appears more black and white)
Edge enhancement	Selective enhancement of the gray scale pixel differences to improve tissue definition

Table 3.1 SELECTED IMAGING GLOSSARY: CARDIAC ULTRASOUND
INSTRUMENTATION "KNOBOLOGY" (continued)

Field of view	FOV; region of interest (ROI) or scan sector width; pie-shaped image with scan sector swivel or sweep angle ±45° (typical range 15° to 90°); see Scan sector; Sector width
Focal zone	See Focus
Focus	Narrowest region of the ultrasound beam that exhibits the best spatial resolution; also called focal zone, focal spot, focal point
Focus, dynamic	Technique for adjusting the focus of an ultrasound beam
Focus number and position	For increasing the number of transmit focal zones or moving the position of the focal zone
FOV	See Field of view; Scan sector; Sector width
Frame	Digital memory of cardiac ultrasound display (typical display is composed of 512 × 512 pixels). Still-frame or freeze-frame of B-mode video display; display scan sector
Frame average	Temporal filter for averaging frames to display an aesthetically smoother image.
Frame rate	The rate or frequency at which the ultrasound equipment can process and display image frames in real-time (frames/sec); ~30 frame/sec processing power needed to display flicker-free images in real time. To increase frame rate: narrow scan sector, decrease imaging depth, and decrease line density.
Freeze	Freeze-frame; still-frame of video image display
Freeze-frame	See Freeze; still-frame
Frequency	See Transducer frequency, Pulse Repetition Frequency (PRP); Multifrequency
Gain	System gain; used to amplify weak echoes and improve image contrast; avoid excessive gain (especially in the operating theatre setting)
Gray map	See Grayscale map
Grayscale map	Scale displayed with B-mode (gray scale) images that indicate echo strength or intensity; structures that produce echoes with the highest intensities appear white (echoreflective, "echobright"); structures that produce few or no echoes appear black (echolucent or "echo free"); the human eye can discern 16 to 32 intermediate shades of gray out of a potentially displayable 256 shades of gray
Harmonic imaging	A technique to improve image quality; selectively uses echoes with harmonic frequencies echoes to create the image; it can reduce artifact and improve image quality
Harmonics	See Harmonic imaging
Image	Reconstruction of the anatomical scan plane to form the scan sector display (image frame) by processing the received echo signals

(continues)

Table 3.1 SELECTED IMAGING GLOSSARY: CARDIAC ULTRASOUND
INSTRUMENTATION "KNOBOLOGY" *(continued)*

Image optimization	Includes: presets, transducer frequency, imaging depth, focal points, gain/TGC, auto-optimize functions
Imaging artifact	*See* Artifact
Keyboard	Input device for entering patient data, annotations, and other entries
Line density	Scan line density; adjust to optimize B-Mode frame rates or spatial resolution; the number of scan lines within scan sector; frame rate, and temporal resolution decreased with increased line density because of finite speed of ultrasound
Log compression	Preprocessing function that compresses the amplitudes of received echo signals using a logarithmic scale; this facilitates improved image display
Mechanical index (MI)	Acoustic output measure to describe the nonthermal and biosafety effects of ultrasound, e.g., cavitation, microbubble rupture; compares two parameters: peak rarefactional pressure and center frequency of the transmitted ultrasound
M-mode	Time-motion-mode (T-M Mode); one-dimensional echocardiography over time with time on the x-axis and depth on the y-axis
Multifrequency	Feature that allows multi-Hertz transducer operation
Multi-Hertz	*See* Multi-frequency
Operator	Instrument operator, sonographer
Optimization	*See* Image Optimization
Probe	Transducer housing, but commonly called the transducer
PRF	*See* Pulse-repetition frequency
Pulse-repetition frequency	Pulse rate or PRF; the number of separate pulses that are sent out every second by the transducer; the pulse-echo operation requires that the transducer must wait for the echoes ("round trip") before transmitting another imaging pulse; PRF typically ranges from 1,000 to 5,000 pulses per second (1–5 kHz); PRF and hence improved frame rates are possible when imaging at shallow depths
Read zoom	A postprocessing function that allows simple image magnification of an operator-defined region of interest within a stored image (no change in image resolution compared to "write zoom")
Region of interest (ROI)	Anatomical area of interest within the ultrasound imaging plane
Rejection	Selection of amplification and processing threshold; removal of unwanted "noise"
RES	Regional expansion selection (*see* Write zoom)
Resolution	Imaging detail; the ability to display image detail without blurring; axial, lateral, slice-thickness, temporal, and contrast resolution

Table 3.1 SELECTED IMAGING GLOSSARY: CARDIAC ULTRASOUND
INSTRUMENTATION "KNOBOLOGY" *(continued)*

Scan line density	*See* Line density
Scan plane	Anatomical scan plane within range of transducer beam
Scan sector	Pie-shaped image frame of anatomical scan plane produced by phased array transducers
Sector scan	*See* Scan sector
Sector size	*See* Sector width; Field of view (FOV); scan angle plus image depth
Sector width	Pie-shaped image with scan sector sweep angle ±45°; a wide scan sector (with increased line density) results in lower frame rates and temporal resolution
Smoothing	Image smoothing or softening; a postprocessing function
Spatial compounding	Technique for improving image quality by combining or averaging ultrasound images acquired from multiple insonation angles into a single image
Suppression	Removal of unwanted low-level echoes or acoustic "noise"
Sweep speed	To change speed at which the timeline is swept
TGC	*See* Time gain compensation
Time gain compensation	TGC; compensates for beam attenuation (loss of acoustic energy with increasing imaging depth); depth-dependent amplification of echoes using sliding controls on display panel (apply based on appearance of image display); also called depth gain compensation (DGC), time varied gain, or variable swept gain
Trace	Measurement tool for tracing selected region of interest, e.g., circumferences and cross-sectional areas
Trackball/joystick	Pointing device or computer mouse for controlling multiple operations of the ultrasound system, e.g., position, scroll, measurements, and analyses
Transducer	The probe housing the piezoelectric elements; phased array transducers permit a wide range of view despite confinement to a small transducer "foot print," e.g., the intercostal spaces or the esophageal lumen
Transducer frequency	A fundamental characteristic of the ultrasound beam (measured in megahertz, MHz); for transthoracic and transesophageal echocardiography, typical values range from 2–5 MHz to 5–7.5 MHz, respectively; modern transducers are capable of multihertz operation
Transmit power	*See* Acoustic power
Write zoom	A preprocessing function to allow image magnification of operator-defined region of interest within an active image; improved image resolution achieved by re-scanning of selected region (with increase in line density and pixels compared to "read zoom"); RES: regional expansion selection
Zoom	*See* Read zoom, Write zoom

CREATING THE ULTRASOUND IMAGE
Figure 3.6

The basics of ultrasound image generation.

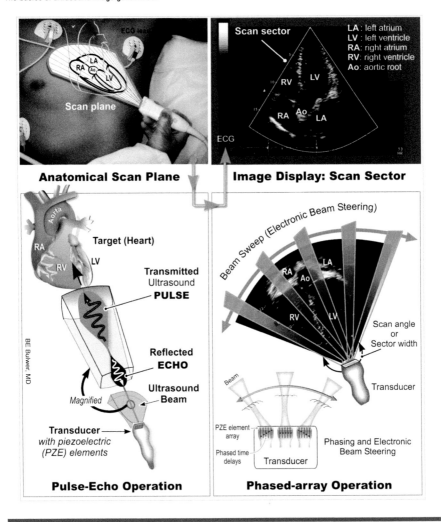

Top panel left. The transducer ultrasound beam scans a defined anatomical region known as the anatomical scan plane. Ultrasound echoes reflected from cardiac structures are processed to generate the image display scan sector.

Bottom panel left. All ultrasound imaging, with the exception of continuous-wave Doppler echocardiography, is based on the pulse-echo method of operation *(left)*. This method uses the return trip times of the reflected echoes to calculate anatomical distances and reconstruct cardiac anatomy. Ultrasound waves or pulses are generated by activation of piezoelectric (PZE) elements housed within the transducer. These highly sensitive components generate ultrasound pulses upon electrical excitation. When ultrasound echoes are received by the transducer, the reverse occurs, and the signals are processed into the ultrasound image display. Analysis of the *round-trip times* and *amplitudes* of the received echoes is the basis of anatomical imaging. Analysis of the *frequency change* or *shift* between the transmitted ultrasound and the received echoes arising from flowing blood or cardiac motion is the basis of Doppler echocardiography. The phased array transducer operation uses electronic phasing or staggered time delays to steer and focus the ultrasound beam *(right)*.

Below right. The phased array transducer operation uses electronic phasing or staggered time delays to steer and focus the ultrasound beam. *Phasing* refers to the capacity to phase or electronically control the timing of PZE element excitation. This is the basis of electronic steering and focusing of the ultrasound beam. The phased array transducer operation used in echocardiography allows the scanning of a wide field of view despite the transducer being confined to the small "footprint" or intercostal space ("window"). The electronic beam steering or sweep through the anatomical scan plane is the basis of generating the image scan sector (*Above right;* Figure 3.11).

THE SOUND SPECTRUM AND MEDICAL ULTRASOUND
Figure 3.7

The sound spectrum and medical ultrasound.

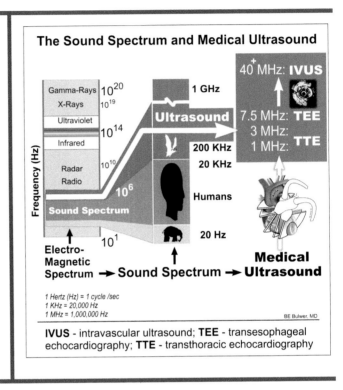

IVUS - intravascular ultrasound; TEE - transesophageal echocardiography; TTE - transthoracic echocardiography

The sound spectrum can be categorized as infrasonic (or subsonic), audible, and ultrasonic. Audible sound exhibits frequencies below 20,000 cycles per second (20×10^3 Hertz, [Hz]) in adults Figure 3.7 . Ultrasound, with frequencies greater than 15 to 20 kHz ($15 \times 10^3 - 20 \times 10^3$ cycles per second), is inaudible. Ultrasound exhibits characteristics that can be harnessed in medical diagnostic imaging. Ultrasound (i) can be directed as a beam, (ii) obeys the laws of reflection and refraction, and (iii) is differentially reflected from cardiac structures, with the returning echoes translated into images.

Ultrasound, however, travels poorly in air. As a result, ultrasonography in general, and transthoracic echocardiography in particular, requires "windows" that avoid or minimize exposure to the air-filled lung. Diagnostic medical ultrasonography uses transducers with frequencies ranging from 2 million Hz to 15 million Hz, or 2 to 15 megahertz (MHz). Newer applications like intravascular ultrasound (IVUS) use frequencies exceeding 40 MHz.

SOUND WAVE CHARACTERISTICS
Figure 3.8

Basic properties of sound waves.

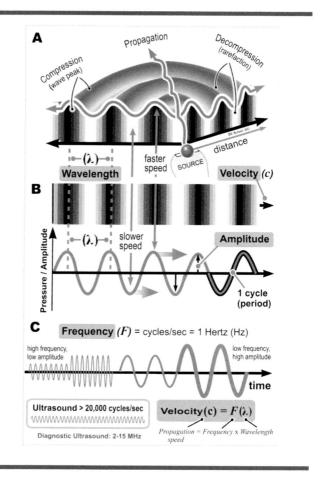

Wavelength, amplitude, velocity, and frequency are important characteristics of ultrasound that influence its usefulness as well as its limitations.

Wavelength and frequency influence the depth of penetration, and hence image quality, resolution (detail), and imaging artifacts.

The *amplitude* of the reflected echoes is the property that determines brightness modulation (B-mode) appearance Figure 3.11 .

Changes in the frequency are used in Doppler echocardiography to determine blood flow velocities, hemodynamics, and cardiac motion. (See Chapter 4.)

The *speed* or *velocity* of ultrasound averages 1,540 m/s in soft tissues, such as those of the heart.

INTERACTIONS OF SOUND WAVES WITH BODY TISSUES

Ultrasound interacts differently with different tissues, and the images we see or don't see portray the nature and the extent of these interactions. The "echoreflectivity" or brightness of the images, image detail, image distortion, and artifact are all related to how ultrasound interacts with tissues.

When ultrasound encounters tissues in its path, e.g., the skin → subcutaneous tissues → chest wall → pleura → lung → pericardium → myocardium → endocardium → blood (Figures 3.9, 3.10), it interacts differentially with each tissue boundary. A portion of the ultrasound is reflected, and the remainder is scattered, refracted, diffracted, and/or attenuated to varying extents as it traverses these tissues.

Reflection is the basis of all ultrasound imaging. It is only the reflected ultrasound (echoes) received by the transducers that participate in image formation. The strongest reflections, i.e., echoes with the largest amplitudes, arise at tissue interfaces (boundaries). The strength of the reflected echoes and the extent to which the ultrasound is reflected depend on:

1. The *angle* of the incident ultrasound beam relative to the target—whether perpendicular or oblique (Figures 3.9, 3.10). Anatomical images are best seen when the ultrasound beam is aligned perpendicular to the imaged target. In contrast, blood flow velocities obtained by Doppler echocardiography are most accurate when the ultrasound beam is aligned parallel to the direction of blood flow.
2. The "*smoothness*" or *size* of the target organ or reflector relative to the *wavelength* of the incident ultrasound beam, whether *specular* (mirror-like) or *nonspecular* (Figures 3.9, 3.10). Ultrasound "sees" images as smooth when the imaged target is bigger than the ultrasound wavelength.
3. The difference in *acoustic impedance* directly influences the degree to which different tissues impede ultrasound transmission (Figure 3.10).

Reflection: When the incident ultrasound beam is perpendicular to a *specular* tissue boundary or interface like the pericardium or pleura, most is reflected directly back along its incident path (Figures 3.9–3.11). This creates strong echoes, i.e., echoes with the largest amplitude spikes on A-mode (Figure 3.11). Such echoes appear as highly *echoreflective* (*hyperechoic* or "*echobright*") structures on B-mode (Figures 3.9–3.11). When the incident beam encounters a relatively rough or *nonspecular* surface, this results in scattering of the beam in multiple directions. The resultant echoes are called *backscatter*. Most backscattered echoes do not directly return to the transducer. However, they generate useful inhomogeneous granular patterns called "speckles." Speckles can serve as tissue "signatures," especially within the myocardium. Tracking the movements of these "signatures" throughout the cardiac cycle is the basis of speckle tracking echocardiography.

Compared to specular reflectors, which produce hyperechoic echoes (that appear white on the echocardiographic image display), nonspecular reflectors produce *hypoechoic* echoes with smaller amplitudes that appear as various shades of gray. This is the basis of B-mode or brightness mode echocardiography. *Anechoic* or *echolucent* structures, which absorb almost all the incident ultrasound beam (i.e., little or no reflection), appear echo free (or black) on the B-mode image display. Tiny scatterers of ultrasound, such as the red blood cells, produce little or no echoes on B-mode. However, useful changes in the frequency—as compared to amplitude—of the returning echoes from moving red blood cells occur. This change in frequency of the echoes is the basis of Doppler echocardiography.

Refraction decribes a change in the direction of a nonperpendicular incident ultrasound beam. This can lead to image distortion and refraction artifacts.

Attenuation refers to the inevitable loss of ultrasound wave amplitude or beam intensity, with distance traveled within the imaged tissue due to absorption and scatter. Attenuation appears as image degradation or image dropout, and are seen in the far field of the ultrasound image display. Attenuation artifact can be reduced by time-gain or depth-gain compensation Figure 3.5 .

Figure 3.9

Schematic summary of interaction of the emitted ultrasound waves with tissues *(top)* and corresponding echocardiographic image display *(bottom)*. When ultrasound encounters tissues in its path, it is reflected, scattered, refracted, diffracted, and attenuated to varying degrees (see Figure 3.10). Processing of the received echoes is the basis of all ultrasound imaging. The types of interactions determine the appearance of ultrasound echoes reflected from various structures. Specular or mirror-like reflectors, e.g., those originating at the pericardium-lung pleura boundary, emit the strongest echoes and appear hyperechoic or "echobright."

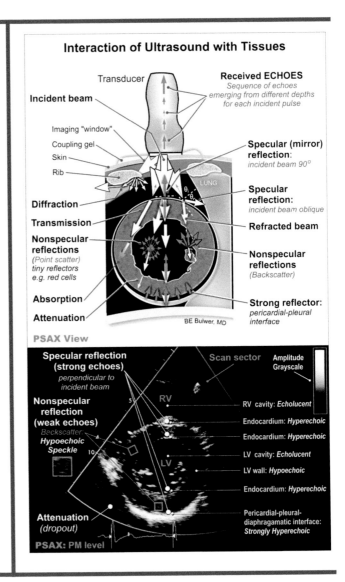

Interaction of Ultrasound with Tissues

Transducer

Incident beam

Received ECHOES
Sequence of echoes emerging from different depths for each incident pulse

Imaging "window"

Coupling gel

Skin

Rib

LUNG

Specular (mirror) reflection:
incident beam 90°

Specular reflection:
incident beam oblique

Diffraction

Transmission

Nonspecular reflections
(Point scatter)
tiny reflectors
e.g. red cells

Refracted beam

Nonspecular reflections
(Backscatter)

Absorption

Attenuation

BE Bulwer, MD

Strong reflector:
pericardial-pleural interface

PSAX View

Specular reflection (strong echoes)
perpendicular to incident beam

Nonspecular reflection (weak echoes)
Backscatter:
Hypoechoic Speckle

Attenuation
(dropout)

Scan sector

Amplitude Grayscale

RV

LV

RV cavity: *Echolucent*

Endocardium: *Hyperechoic*

Endocardium: *Hyperechoic*

LV cavity: *Echolucent*

LV wall: *Hypoechoic*

Endocardium: *Hyperechoic*

Pericardial-pleural-diaphragamatic interface: *Strongly Hyperechoic*

PSAX: PM level

Figure 3.10

Tabular summary of the interaction of ultrasound with tissues.

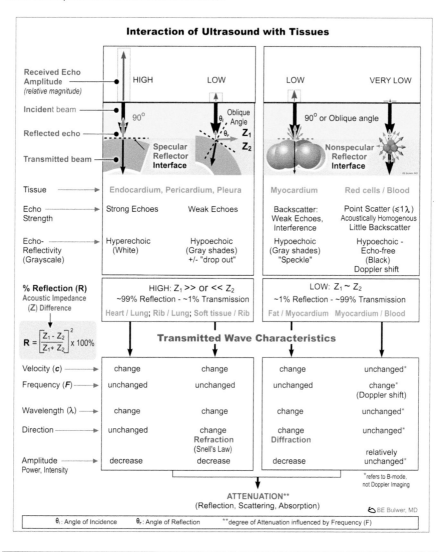

Interaction of Ultrasound with Tissues

Received Echo Amplitude (relative magnitude)	HIGH	LOW	LOW	VERY LOW
		Specular Reflector Interface	Nonspecular Reflector Interface	
Tissue	Endocardium, Pericardium, Pleura		Myocardium	Red cells / Blood
Echo Strength	Strong Echoes	Weak Echoes	Backscatter: Weak Echoes, Interference	Point Scatter ($\leq 1\lambda$) Acoustically Homogenous Little Backscatter
Echo-Reflectivity (Grayscale)	Hyperechoic (White)	Hypoechoic (Gray shades) +/- "drop out"	Hypoechoic (Gray shades) "Speckle"	Hypoechoic - Echo-free (Black) Doppler shift
% Reflection (R) Acoustic Impedance (Z) Difference	HIGH: $Z_1 \gg$ or $\ll Z_2$ ~99% Reflection - ~1% Transmission Heart / Lung; Rib / Lung; Soft tissue / Rib		LOW: $Z_1 \sim Z_2$ ~1% Reflection - ~99% Transmission Fat / Myocardium Myocardium / Blood	

$$R = \left[\frac{Z_1 - Z_2}{Z_1 + Z_2} \right]^2 \times 100\%$$

Transmitted Wave Characteristics

Velocity (c)	change	change	change	unchanged*
Frequency (F)	unchanged	unchanged	unchanged	change* (Doppler shift)
Wavelength (λ)	change	change	change	unchanged*
Direction	unchanged	change Refraction (Snell's Law)	change Diffraction	unchanged*
Amplitude Power, Intensity	decrease	decrease	decrease	relatively unchanged*

*refers to B-mode, not Doppler Imaging

ATTENUATION**
(Reflection, Scattering, Absorption)

🔷 BE Bulwer, MD

θ_i: Angle of Incidence θ_r: Angle of Reflection   **degree of Attenuation influenced by Frequency (F)

GENERATION OF A-MODE AND B-MODE IMAGES
Figure 3.11

Upper left. Scan plane anatomy (PSAX, parasternal short-axis view), scan lines, and echo signals received by the transducer from various depths. Ultrasound travels at speeds averaging 1,540 meters/sec (1.54 mm/İsec). The phased array transducer beam rapidly sweeps through multiple scan lines. *Upper right.* Processing the amplitudes of echoes returning from various depths can be graphically depicted on an amplitude-modulated (A-mode) oscilloscope display—a format no longer used in echocardiography. Brightness-modulation (B-mode) displays using shades of gray (or gray scale) is the standard used in echocardiography. This B-mode information can be displayed using a one-dimensional "ice-pick view" over time using a motion-mode (M-mode) format (lower right), on two-dimensions as a (2D) or cross-sectional image *(lower left),* or in three dimensions (3D).

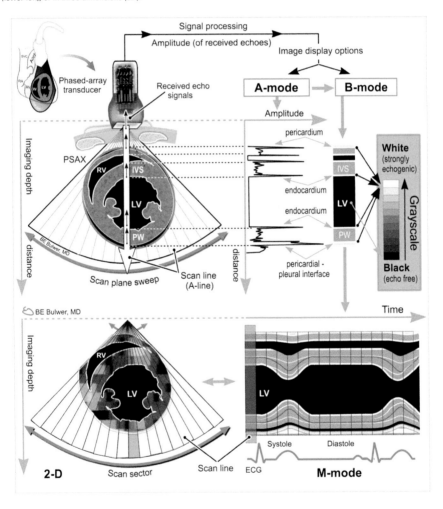

B-MODE IMAGE DISPLAY OPTIONS
Figure 3.12

Schematic of the parasternal long-axis (PLAX) view showing B-mode image display options. The basis of the B- (bright-ness) mode display is that the amplitude of the echoes arising from the imaged structure are processed and displayed in grayscale. *Echolucent* or *anechoic* components, e.g., blood and serous fluids, appear black. Highly reflective (*hyper-echoic* or *strongly echogenic*) structures, e.g., pericardium/pleural surfaces and calcified tissues, appear white. Struc-tures of intermediate echoreflectivity e.g., the myocardium, appear heterogenous or as speckled shades of gray. B-mode images can be displayed using one- (1D), two- (2D), or three-dimensional (3D) formats. The M-mode display format, be-cause of its excellent temporal resolution, remains useful for the timing of fast-moving structures, e.g., heart valves. It was the original display format. 2D is the standard cross-sectional display format, with real-time 3D displays being the most re-cent option. *aml: anterior mitral leaflet; pml: posterior mitral leaflet.*

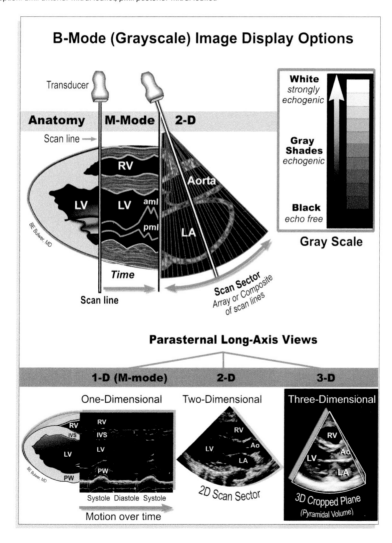

B-MODE IMAGE FREEZE FRAMES
Figure 3.13

A still- or freeze-frame of the 2D cross-sectional image display. Note the presence and significance of various parameters and instrument settings that influence the appearance and quality of the 2D image display.

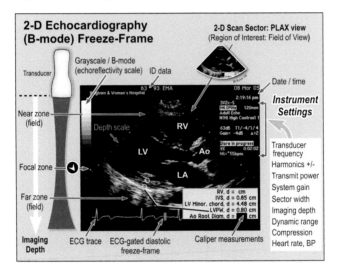

Figure 3.14

A still- or freeze-frame of the M-mode image display. Note the parameters and instrument settings that influence the appearance and quality of the M-mode display.

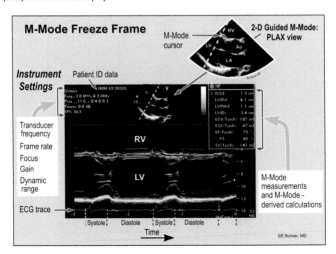

CHAPTER 4

Blood Flow Hemodynamics, Cardiac Mechanics, and Doppler Echocardiography

THE CARDIAC CYCLE
Figure 4.1

The cardiac cycle showing superimposed hemodynamic and echocardiographic parameters. *A4C: apical 4-chamber view; A5C: apical 5-chamber view; AC: aortic valve closure; AO: aortic valve opening; E- and A-waves: spectral Doppler depiction of early and late diastolic filling of the left ventricle; MC: mitral valve closure; MO: mitral valve opening; LA: left atrium; LV: left ventricle; left atrial "a" and "e" waves reflecting atrial pressures; EDV: end diastolic LV volume; ESV: end-systolic LV volume.*

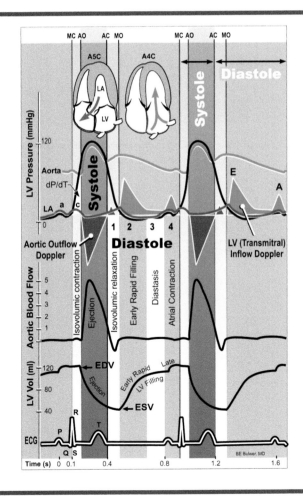

Figure 4.2

Flow velocity profiles in normal pulsatile blood flow. Normal blood flow through the heart and blood vessels, at any instant in time, is not uniform. There is a range or spectrum of velocities at each instant during the cardiac cycle. This spectrum, at each instant during the cardiac cycle, can be differentiated and displayed using Doppler echocardiography (see Figures 4.3–4.22).

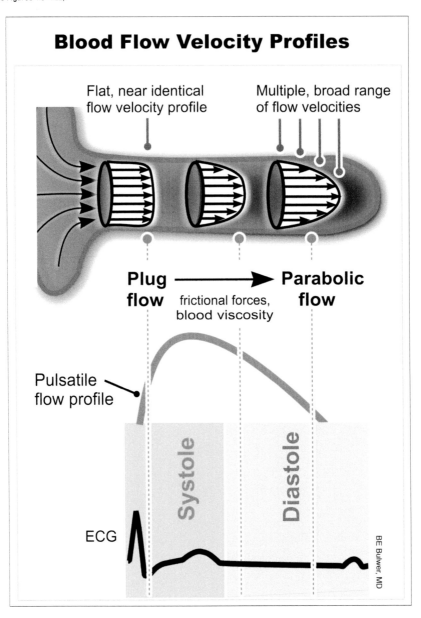

BLOOD FLOW VELOCITY PROFILES

Doppler echocardiography can assess blood flow velocity, direction and flow patterns/profiles (e.g., plug), and laminar, parabolic, and turbulent flow Figures 4.3–4.19 . Crucial to understanding Doppler echocardiography is the need to understand certain basic characteristics of blood flow. Blood vessel size, shape, wall characteristics, flow rate, phase of the cardiac cycle, and blood viscosity all influence blood flow velocity profiles. Even within the cross-sectional area of a blood vessel, there exists a differential pattern of flow.

The range or spectrum of blood flow velocities widens or broadens at sites of blood vessel narrowing and near stenotic or regurgitant heart valves Figures 4.7, 4.14, 4.15 . Even within the normal heart and blood vessels, various blood flow velocity profiles are seen as vessels curve around valve orifices Figures 4.7, 4.9, 4.14, 4.15, 4.17–4.19 . Normal blood flow through the heart, however, is mostly *laminar* or streamlined, but exhibits *turbulence* or disorganized flow in the presence of diseased heart valves.

Laminar flow within cardiac chambers and great arteries generally exhibits an initial flat or *plug flow* profile during the initial systolic cardiac upstroke Figures 4.2, 4.17, 4.19 . With plug flow, almost all of the blood cells (within the sample volume) are flowing at the same velocity. On the time-velocity spectral Doppler display, this appears as a narrow band or range of velocities.

As blood flow proceeds, the velocity flow profile becomes more *parabolic,* especially within long straight vessels like the descending thoracic and abdominal aortae. With laminar flow, concentric streamlines (laminae) glide smoothly along the blood vessel. Laminar flow with a parabolic flow profile exhibits the highest (maximum) velocities at the axial center of the vessel Figures 4.2, 4.17 . Velocities are lowest, approaching zero, adjacent to the vessel wall.

Turbulent flow is disorganized blood flow and exhibits the widest range of flow velocities, including high-velocity and multidirectional flow Figures 4.7, 4.14, 4.15 . Turbulent flow is typically seen with obstructive and regurgitant valvular lesions, prosthetic heart valves, shunts, and arteriovenous fistulae Figures 4.7, 4.14, 4.15 .

NORMAL BLOOD FLOW THROUGH THE HEART
Figure 4.3

Normal blood flow patterns through the heart (anteropostero projections). Right-sided deoxygenated flows returning to the heart en route to the lungs are shown in blue. Oxygenated flows returning to the heart from the lungs are shown in red. Isolated right and left heart flow patterns are shown below.

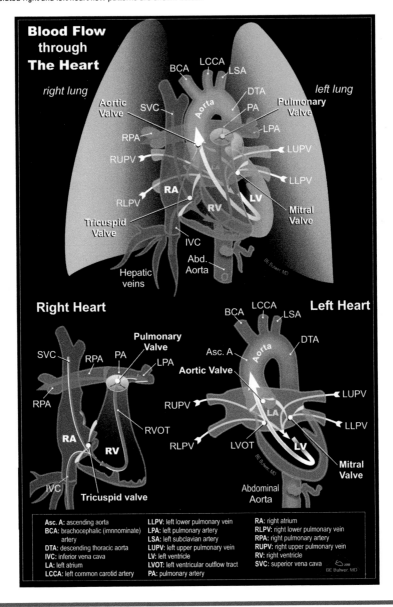

Asc. A: ascending aorta	**LLPV:** left lower pulmonary vein	**RA:** right atrium
BCA: brachocephalic (imnnominate) artery	**LPA:** left pulmonary artery	**RLPV:** right lower pulmonary vein
	LSA: left subclavian artery	**RPA:** right pulmonary artery
DTA: descending thoracic aorta	**LUPV:** left upper pulmonary vein	**RUPV:** right upper pulmonary vein
IVC: inferior vena cava	**LV:** left ventricle	**RV:** right ventricle
LA: left atrium	**LVOT:** left ventricular outflow tract	**SVC:** superior vena cava
LCCA: left common carotid artery	**PA:** pulmonary artery	

DOPPLER INTERROGATION SITES
Figure 4.4

Doppler echocardiography, both color flow Doppler and spectral Doppler, provides accurate noninvasive assessment of normal and abnormal intracardiac blood flow, and flow across the heart valves. *AV: aortic valve; DTA: descenders thoracic aortia; IVC: inferior vena cava; LVOT: left ventricular outflow tract; LA: left atrium; LV: left ventricle; MV: mitral valve; PV: pulmonary valve; RVOT: right ventricular outflow tract; TV: tricuspid valve.*

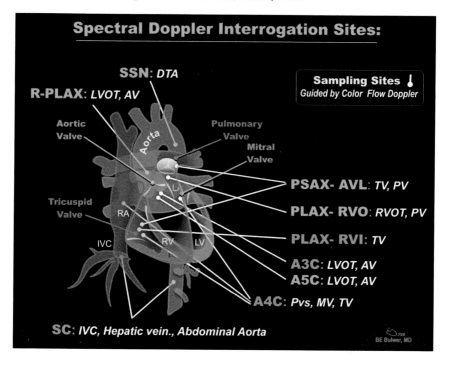

Assessment of blood flow velocities and flow patterns, made possible by Doppler echocardiography, are a routine part of the normal echocardiography examination. Two basic types of Doppler displays are used to assess blood flow velocities: the spectral Doppler time-velocity graph and color flow Doppler map Figures 1.1, 4.6, 4.7, 4.12, 4.13, 4.16, 4.21.

The spectral Doppler time-velocity graph displays the spectrum of blood flow velocities found within the sample volume. The sample volume is the specified region interrogated during the Doppler exam. It ranges from a few millimeters in length (with pulsed-wave [PW] Doppler), to several centimeters in length (as with continuous-wave [CW] Doppler). CW Doppler is used to assess high-flow velocities, but lacks depth specificity, i.e., CW Doppler can measure the highest velocities, but it cannot accurately pinpoint the exact location where such high blood velocities occur. PW Doppler echocardiography, in contrast, measures flow at specific sites, but it is handicapped by a measurement artifact called *aliasing* that imposes a limit *(Nyquisit limit)* on the maximum measurable velocity. Aliased velocities erroneously appear on the opposite side of the baseline Figure 4.22 .

Color flow Doppler imaging is a PW Doppler-based technique that displays blood flow velocities as real-time color flow patterns mapped within the cardiac chambers Figures 4.9–4.13 . Conceptually, this can be considered as a type of "color angiogram." By convention, color flow Doppler velocities are displayed using the "BART" (Blue Away Red Toward) scale Figures 4.9–4.11 . Flow toward the transducer is color-coded red; flow away from the transducer is color-coded blue. Color flow Doppler is beset by the same flow velocity measurement limitations called *color aliasing.* This occurs even at normal intracardiac flow rates. In this case, however, aliasing appears as a color inversion, where flow blue switches to yellow-red, and vice versa Figure 4.22 . Turbulent flow appears as a mosaic of colors.

NORMAL INTRACARDIAC PRESSURES

Figure 4.5

Doppler echocardiography is an accurate noninvasive alternative to cardiac catheterization for estimating blood flow hemodynamics, intracardiac pressures, and valvular function. The relationship between blood flow velocities and intracardiac pressures is quantitatively defined by the Bernoulli equation (see Figure 4.14).

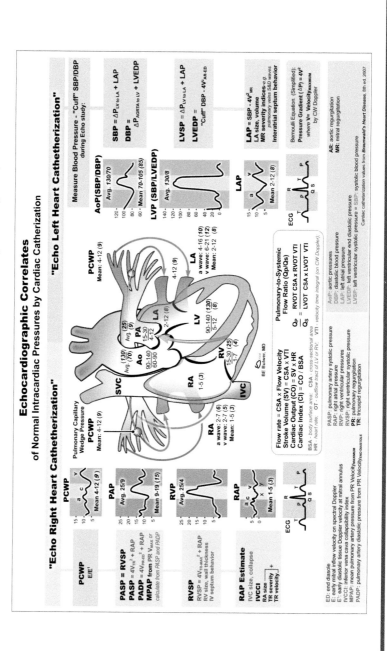

Echocardiographic Correlates
of Normal Intracardiac Pressures by Cardiac Catheterization

DOPPLER FREQUENCY SHIFT
Figure 4.6

The Doppler frequency shift is a change or *shift* in the *frequency* of the returning echoes compared to the frequency of transmitted ultrasound waves. *Top panel.* When blood flows toward the transducer, the received echoes return at higher frequencies compared to the transmitted ultrasound—a positive frequency shift. *Bottom panel.* When blood flows away from the transducer, the converse is seen. *Central panel.* Doppler echocardiography uses this observed and measurable change in frequency—the Doppler frequency shift—to derive information on blood flow velocity and direction *(see Figure 4.7).* The Doppler frequency shift is itself a wave, with its own frequency characteristics.

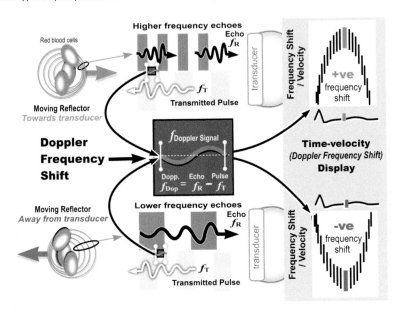

The shift in frequency of the received echoes compared to that of the transmitted pulse—the Doppler frequency shift—is the basis for calculating blood flow velocities.

- **Negative frequency shift:** Echoes reflected from blood flowing away from the transducer have lower frequencies, compared to the transmitted ultrasound Figures 4.6, 4.7 .
- **Positive frequency shift:** Echoes reflected from blood flowing toward the transducer have higher frequencies, compared to the transmitted ultrasound Figures 4.6, 4.7 .
- **No frequency shift:** Echoes reflected from blood flowing perpendicular to the transducer exhibit no change in frequency, compared to the transmitted ultrasound Figure 4.7 .

Doppler Frequency Shift $(F_{Doppler}) = F_{Echo} - F_{Transducer\ Pulse}$

Figure 4.7

Simplified schema of the Doppler examination of flow velocities within the thoracic aorta as viewed from the suprasternal notch window. *Left column.* Note (blue) flow in the descending thoracic aorta away from the transducer, the associated negative Doppler frequency shift, and corresponding time-velocity spectral display below the baseline. *Center.* Doppler examination of (red) flow in the ascending aorta shows just the opposite pattern—a positive Doppler frequency shift with velocities displayed above the baseline. *Right column.* During turbulent flow, as in aortic stenosis, higher velocities and a wider range of velocities is evident. Note the broadening of the spectral Doppler time-velocity display—a reflection of a wider range of velocities—appears as a "filled-in" window. Compare with Figure 4.9.

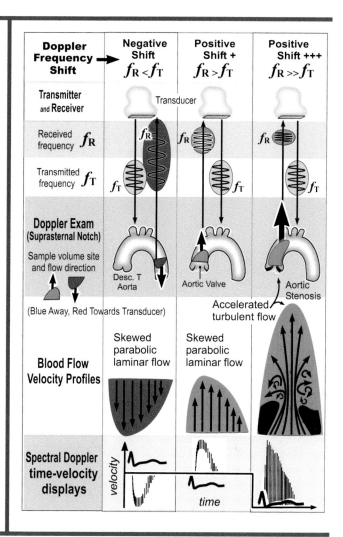

Figure 4.8

The Doppler angle and the Doppler equation. Doppler assessment of blood flow velocities is most accurate when the transducer ultrasound beam is at a Doppler angle of 0° or 180°, i.e., when aligned parallel to blood flow direction. The larger the Doppler angle or the less parallel the alignment, the greater will be the underestimate of true blood flow velocity.

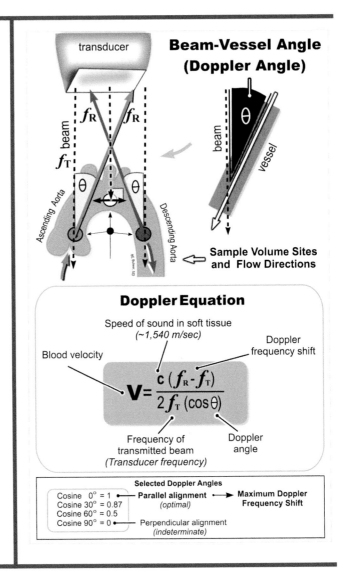

Figure 4.9

Color flow Doppler patterns viewed from the suprasternal notch. Note the flow velocity patterns based on the conventional "BART" (Blue Away Red Toward) scale. Compare this with Figures 4.7, 4.10–4.12. Although the above image shows a wide-angle color scan sector (that covers the entire aortic arch), a narrow color scan sector (that focuses on a narrower region) is recommended. To optimize the color flow Doppler recording: (i) narrow the scan sector, (ii) image at shallower depths (i.e., more superficial structures), (iii) optimize color gain settings, and (iv) set color velocity scale at maximum allowed Nyquist limit for any given depth (generally 60–80 m/s).

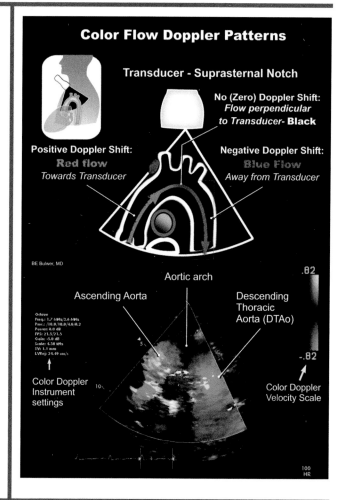

Color Flow Doppler Patterns

Transducer - Suprasternal Notch

No (Zero) Doppler Shift:
Flow perpendicular to Transducer- **Black**

Positive Doppler Shift:
Red flow
Towards Transducer

Negative Doppler Shift:
Blue Flow
Away from Transducer

BE Bulwer, MD

Aortic arch

Ascending Aorta

Descending Thoracic Aorta (DTAo)

.82

Octave
Freq.: 1.7 MHz/3.6 MHz
Pan.: /10.0/10.0/4.0/0.2
Power: 0.0 dB
FPS: 21.5/21.5
Gain: -5.0 dB
Scale: 6.50 kHz
SV: 1.1 mm
LVRej: 24.49 cm/s

-.82

Color Doppler
Instrument
settings

Color Doppler
Velocity Scale

100
HR

CLINICAL UTILITY OF COLOR FLOW DOPPLER ECHOCARDIOGRAPHY

Color flow Doppler imaging provides information on blood flow direction, velocity, and flow patterns, e.g., laminar versus turbulent flow, by displaying blood flow as color-coded velocities superimposed in real time on the 2D or M-mode image Figures 4.9, 4.10 .

This "angiographic" display is a more intuitive depiction of blood flow velocities, and it is extremely useful for the preliminary assessment of blood flow characteristics during the examination. For this reason, color flow Doppler imaging is the initial Doppler modality to use when interrogating flows within cardiac chambers and across valves, and it serves as an important guide for subsequent placement of the sample volume during PW and CW Doppler examination Figure 4.16 .

Figure 4.10

Color flow Doppler convention "BART" scale: Blue Away, Red Toward. Apical four-chamber (A4C) view showing the color flow Doppler map superimposed on a B-mode 2D image. Flow direction during early systole reveals (blue) flow along the left ventricular outflow tract moving away from the transducer. The red color flow indicates flow toward the apex of the left ventricle, i.e., toward the transducer.

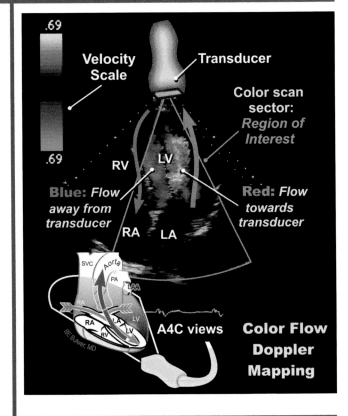

COLOR FLOW DOPPLER VELOCITY AND VARIANCE SCALES
Figure 4.11

Color Doppler scales are velocity reference maps. The standard red-blue velocity "BART" scale *(left)*, the variance scale *(center)*, and the color wheel *(right)* depicting the concept of color aliasing (wrap around) are shown. Variance maps employ an additional color, usually green, to emphasize the wider spectrum of multidirectional velocities present during turbulent flow.

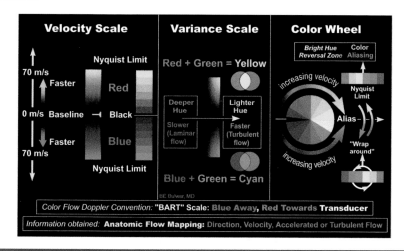

Figure 4.12

Color flow Doppler freeze frame showing components, variables, and instrument settings.

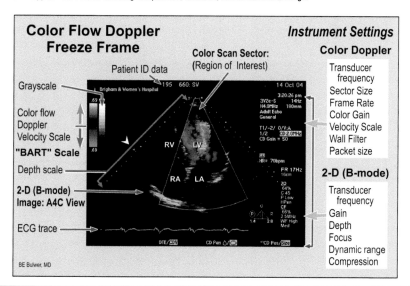

INSTRUMENT SETTINGS INFLUENCING COLOR FLOW DOPPLER IMAGING AND DISPLAY

Main factors (Figures 4.12, 4.13, 4.22):

- **Transmit power:** acoustic power output
- **Color gain setting:** amplifies the strength of the color velocities; avoid too much or too little gain
- **Transducer frequency:** trade-off between image resolution and tissue penetration; influences color jet size (for example, in mitral regurgitation)
- **Color velocity scale, Pulse-repetition frequency (PRF):** higher PRFs reduce aliasing but reduce sensitivity to low-flow velocities; lower PRFs increase the sensitivity to detect lower-flow velocities, but increase aliasing
- **Baseline shift:** determines range of color velocities displayed in a particular direction on the color velocity scale. This adjustment is also necessary for the assessment of the severity of valvular regurgitation and stenosesusing the proximal isovelocity surface area (PISA) method (see Chapter 6, Figures 6.25, 6.26).
- **Color scan sector size:** improved frame rate and hence color display quality with narrow color scan sector
- **Packet (burst, ensemble) size and line density:** set at medium—a trade-off between measurement accuracy, image resolution, and frame rate
- **Focus:** color flow imaging is optimal at the focal zone

Other factors:

- **Persistence (smoothing, temporal filtering):** a higher setting delivers a smoother image, but lowers image resolution
- **Wall filter (threshold/high-pass filter):** this setting reduces artifacts due to vessel wall motion

COLOR FLOW DOPPLER EXAMINATION SUMMARY
Figure 4.13

Summary chart of the color flow Doppler examination. The color flow Doppler exam is an integral part of the standard transthoracic examination (see Table 5.4, Figures 4.21 and 5.4). As outlined in the standard transthoracic examination protocol, color flow Doppler is used to interrogate specific heart valves and chambers after optimizing the 2D image. Color flow Doppler-guided pulsed wave (PW) and continuous-wave (CW) Doppler examination typically follow.

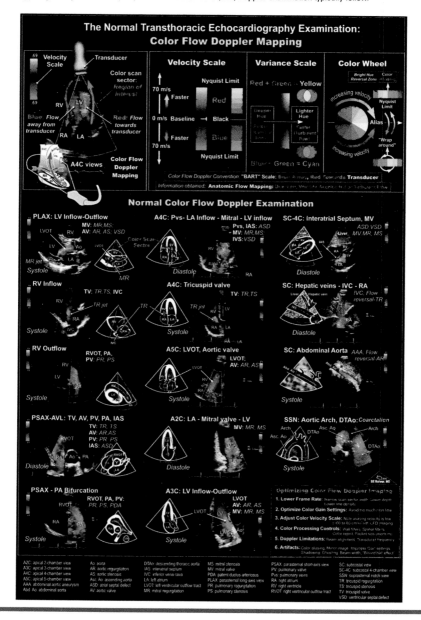

OPTIMIZING COLOR FLOW DOPPLER CONTROLS

Modern echocardiography instruments have important controls for optimizing the color flow Doppler examination Figures 3.4, 4.12 . Each laboratory should implement internal standards that conform to the recommended instrument settings guidelines.

In general, the following practical steps to optimize color flow Doppler imaging should be employed as the transthoracic examination proceeds.

- **Optimize the 2D (or M-mode) image for optimal Doppler beam alignment:** Color Doppler, like all other Doppler techniques, is angle dependent. Parallel alignment is required for optimal color velocity assessment. The region of interest should therefore be optimally aligned Figures 4.10, 4.12, 4.13 .

- **Activate color flow Doppler imaging mode:** On/off knob or switch. During the transthoracic examination, the normal sequence is to (i) optimize the 2D image, (ii) apply color Doppler imaging, and (iii) use the color flow display as a guide to spectral (PW, CW) Doppler sample volume placement Figure 4.16 .

- **Use the narrowest color scan sector (smallest color window):** In general, the active color window or scan sector should be made as small as is necessary to increase frame rate, reduce aliasing, minimize artifact error, and improve overall color resolution/sensitivity Figures 4.10, 4.12 .

- **Adjust color gain control:** The color gain setting is a major determinant of the appearance of the color Doppler flow. Too little color gain can cause the jet to appear smaller or disappear altogether. Excessive gain can cause the jet to appear much larger, thereby overestimating, for example, the valvular regurgitation severity. To optimize this setting, increase the color gain until color pixels start "bleeding" into the B-mode (grayscale) tissue. Stop increasing at this point, then slightly reduce color gain to eliminate such "bleeding."

- **Color velocity scale/pulse-repetition frequency (PRF):** Lowering the velocity scale, i.e., lowering the PRF, enables the detection of lower velocities and hence a larger color jet, but the tradeoff is increased color aliasing. Increasing the velocity scale, i.e., at a higher PRF, reduces color aliasing, but results in a smaller jet. Aliasing on color flow Doppler manifests as "color inversion" or "wrap around" Figures 4.11, 4.22 .

PRESSURE-VELOCITY RELATIONSHIP: THE BERNOULLI EQUATION
Figure 4.14

The velocity of flow across a fixed orifice, e.g., a stenotic heart valve, depends on the pressure gradient or difference (ΔP, "driving pressure") across that orifice. The Bernoulli principle and equation describes this relationship. It serves as the basis of converting blood flow velocities measured by Doppler into intracardiac pressures and pressure gradients. When the proximal velocity (V_1) is significantly smaller (and ~1 m/s) than the distal velocity (V_2), the former can be ignored and the simplified form ($P = 4V^2$) is used. $P = $ intracardiac pressure gradient and $V = $ blood flow velocity. $\rho = $ mass density of blood.

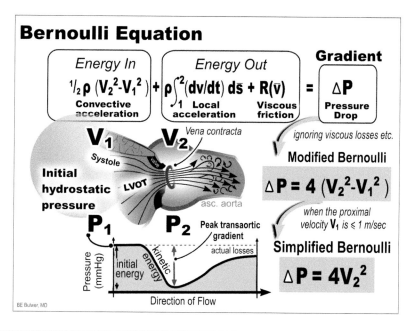

Table 4.1 NORMAL INTRACARDIAC BLOOD VELOCITIES (M/SEC) AND DOPPLER MEASUREMENT SITES

Valve/vessel	Mean	Range	Echo windows/views
Mitral valve	0.90	0.6–1.3	A4C, A2C, A3C
LVOT	0.90	0.7–1.1	A5C, R-PLAX
Aorta	1.35	1.0–1.7	A5C, SSN
Tricuspid valve	0.50	0.3–0.7	RV inflow, PSAX-AVL, A4C
Pulmonary artery	0.75	0.6–0.9	RV outflow, PSAX-AVL

Source: Adapted from: Hatle L, Angelsen B. Doppler *Ultrasound in Cardiology: Physical Principles and Clinical Applications,* 2nd ed. Philadelphia: Lea & Febiger, 1985.

Figure 4.15

The continuity principle applied to the calculation of valve area in aortic valvular stenosis. The calculation of proximal isovelocity surface area (PISA) in valvular heart disease, particularly in mitral regurgitation, is another widely used application of the continuity equation. *A5C: apical 5-chamber view; LVOT: left ventricular outflow tract.*

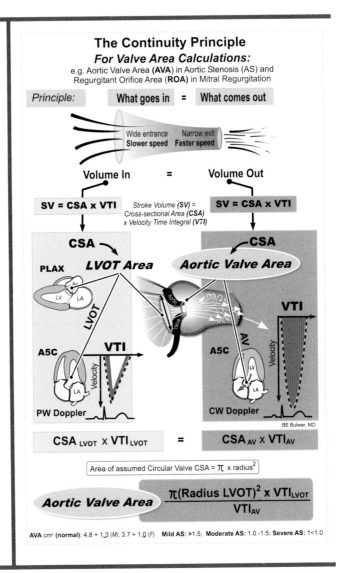

The Continuity Principle
For Valve Area Calculations:
e.g. Aortic Valve Area (**AVA**) in Aortic Stenosis (AS) and Regurgitant Orifice Area (**ROA**) in Mitral Regurgitation

Principle: What goes in = What comes out

Wide entrance Narrow exit
Slower speed Faster speed

Volume In = **Volume Out**

SV = CSA x VTI   Stroke Volume (*SV*) = Cross-sectional Area (*CSA*) x Velocity Time Integral (*VTI*)   **SV = CSA x VTI**

CSA **LVOT Area**   **Aortic Valve Area** **CSA**

PLAX

A5C **VTI**   A5C **VTI**

PW Doppler   CW Doppler

BE Bulwer, MD

$$CSA_{LVOT} \times VTI_{LVOT} = CSA_{AV} \times VTI_{AV}$$

Area of assumed Circular Valve CSA = $\pi \times radius^2$

Aortic Valve Area $\dfrac{\pi(Radius\ LVOT)^2 \times VTI_{LVOT}}{VTI_{AV}}$

AVA *cm²* (normal): 4.8 + 1.3 (*M*); 3.7 + 1.0 (*F*)   **Mild AS:** >1.5; **Moderate AS:** 1.0 -1.5; **Severe AS:** 1<1.0

GRAPHICAL DISPLAY OF DOPPLER FREQUENCY SPECTRA

To generate the spectral Doppler display (Figures 4.6, 4.16–4.21), the received raw echo signals must be processed to extract the Doppler frequency shifts, from which are derived blood flow velocities.

Like a prism that separates white light into its spectral colors, and the cochlea that separates audible sounds into its spectrum of frequencies, so must the raw Doppler data be transformed into a spectrum of Doppler frequency shifts (that correspond to blood flow velocities (Figure 4.2)). This is achieved using a computational analysis called the fast Fourier transformation. Within each vertical spectral band, there is a range of Doppler frequency shifts—maximum and minimum—that corresponds to the range of velocities present within the sample volume at each measured instant in time (Figure 4.18). This range or spectral band is narrow, or broad, depending on the range of flow velocities found within the sampled blood volume. How narrow, or how broad this band is, is a reflection of the blood flow profile—whether plug, or parabolic, or turbulent (Figures 4.7, 4.15, 4.17–4.20).

A plot of Doppler frequency spectra displayed in real time during the cardiac cycle generates the time-velocity spectral Doppler display, variously called the Doppler velocity profile, envelope, or flow signal (Figures 4.16–4.22). Therefore, time-velocity spectral Doppler display reveals a number of important characteristics about the interrogated blood flow:

1. **The range or spectral band of Doppler frequency shifts:** These correspond to the range of blood flow velocities within the sample volume at each instant during the cardiac cycle. The spectral distribution of Doppler shifts at a given instant in time is a measure of flow characteristics, e.g., plug versus parabolic or turbulent flow patterns. With PW Doppler, plug flow (during the early systolic upstroke) exhibits a narrow range or spectrum of Doppler frequency shifts, which manifests as a narrow spectral band with a resultant spectral "window" (Figures 4.6, 4.16–4.22). In later systole, and during diastole, this spectral band broadens due to laminar parabolic flow, i.e., blood with a broader range of velocities. Turbulent flow exhibit the widest range of velocities—regardless of the phase of the cardiac cycle—and appear as broad spectral bands (spectral broadening) with a "filled-in" spectral window on PW Doppler. The Doppler window is characteristically absent or filled-in on the CW Doppler display. This reflects the wide range of velocities normally found within the large CW Doppler sample volume (Figures 4.20–4.22).

2. **Positive, negative, or no Doppler frequency shift:** This indicates the presence and the direction of blood flow (Figures 4.6–4.22). Positive shifts are displayed above the baseline, and they are indicative of flow toward the

transducer. Negative shifts are displayed below the baseline, indicating flow away from the transducer Figures 4.6–4.10 . No measured Doppler shifts, or zero flow, results when the Doppler angle is 90°, or when flow is absent, or the sample volume is beyond the range of the transducer.

3. **The amplitude of the Doppler frequency shifts:** This is apparent from the intensity or brightness of the Doppler display, and corresponds to the percentage of blood cells exhibiting a specific frequency within the individual (vertical) Doppler spectral band Figures 4.17–4.20 .

The Doppler frequency shifts are also within the audible range (0–20 kHz), and such audio signals can guide Doppler sample volume placement, especially when using the dedicated nonimaging (pencil or Pedoff) Doppler probe.

Figure 4.16

The PW Doppler spectral display showing normal mitral inflow (left ventricular filling) patterns obtained from the apical 4-chamber (A4C) view. With PW Doppler imaging, optimal information is derived when close attention is paid to proper technique, including optimal transducer alignment (Doppler angle), as well as the appropriate instrument settings (see Table 4.2).

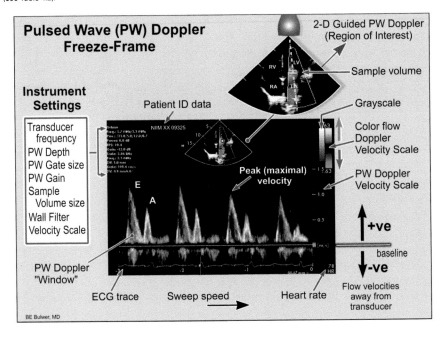

PULSED DOPPLER VELOCITY PROFILE: LEFT VENTRICULAR (TRANSMITRAL) INFLOW
Figure 4.17

Normal transmitral left ventricular inflow: velocity profile and Doppler patterns. During early diastole (1), early rapid inflow exhibits "plug" laminar flow pattern where blood cells are moving en masse at almost the same velocity—hence a narrow spectrum is seen on the pulsed wave (PW) Doppler spectral display. As diastole proceeds (2), a more parabolic laminar low profile ensues where a much broader range of flow velocities—and hence a broader spectrum—is seen. Note the corresponding color flow Doppler patterns (with color-coded mean flow velocities).

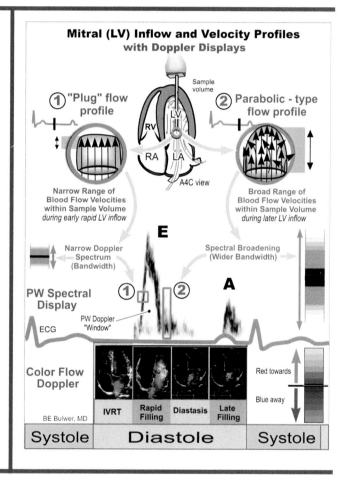

Mitral (LV) Inflow and Velocity Profiles with Doppler Displays

① "Plug" flow profile

② Parabolic - type flow profile

Sample volume

LV
RV
RA LA
A4C view

Narrow Range of Blood Flow Velocities within Sample Volume *during early rapid LV inflow*

Broad Range of Blood Flow Velocities within Sample Volume *during later LV inflow*

E

Narrow Doppler Spectrum (Bandwidth)

Spectral Broadening (Wider Bandwidth)

A

PW Spectral Display

① ②

PW Doppler "Window"

ECG

Color Flow Doppler

BE Bulwer, MD

Red towards

Blue away

| IVRT | Rapid Filling | Diastasis | Late Filling |

Systole   Diastole   Systole

PW DOPPLER AND VELOCITY PROFILE: MEAN AND MAXIMUM VELOCITIES
Figure 4.18

Pulsed-wave (PW) Doppler spectral display of the transmitral LV inflow (compare with Figure 4.17). *Above, from left to right:* Closer scrutiny of the spectral Doppler display reveals vertical bands (spectra) representing the Doppler frequency shifts/blood flow velocities at each measured instant in time (milliseconds). Each vertical spectral band shows the range of velocities—maximum and minimum—present in each measurement. This spectral band is narrow, or broad, depending on the range of flow velocities found within the sampled blood volume. How narrow, or how broad this band is, is a reflection on the blood flow profile—whether plug, or parabolic, or turbulent. E and A waves represent early and late diastolic filling, respectively. *Below:* Doppler-derived blood flow velocities can be converted into pressure gradients using the Bernoulli equation (see Figure 4.14).

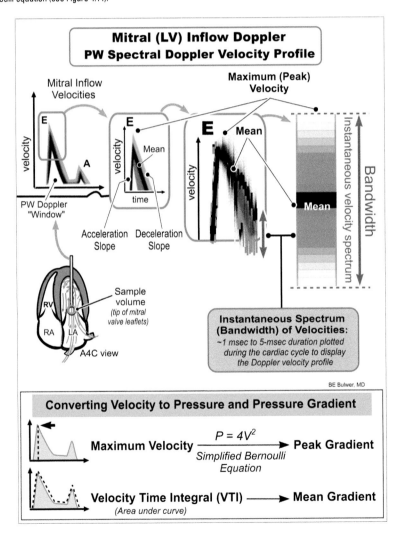

PULSED DOPPLER VELOCITY PROFILE: LEFT VENTRICULAR OUTFLOW
Figure 4.19

Simplified schema of flow velocity profiles and corresponding pulsed-wave Doppler display in the ascending aorta as measured from the apical 5-chamber (A5C) view. **1.** During early ejection, plug flow predominates—and hence a narrow spectrum or range of flow velocities is seen on the spectral display. **2 and 3.** As systole ensues, drag forces contribute to a more parabolic type flow profile with a wider spectrum of velocities. **4.** During late systole, some amount of backflow occurs within the ascending aorta. This manifests as "positive" (above the baseline) flow and results in aortic valve closure.

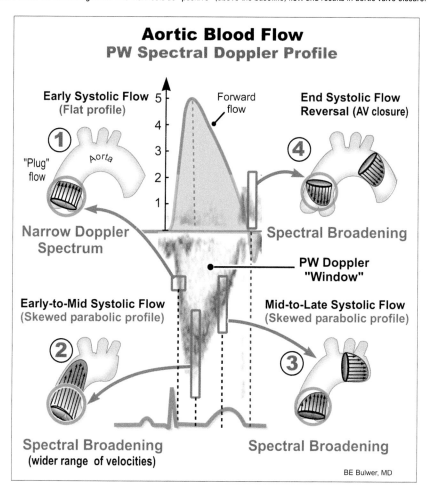

BE Bulwer, MD

CONTINUOUS-WAVE (CW) DOPPLER: PEAK AND MEAN VELOCITIES AND GRADIENTS
Figure 4.20

Continuous-wave (CW) spectral Doppler display of the aortic outflow using the apical 5-chamber view. Note the wide spectrum of frequencies/velocities that broaden the Doppler frequency spectrum. Compared to the PW Doppler display (Figure 4.19, the CW spectral displays show spectral broadening with a "filled-in" Doppler window). This is a reflection of the large CW Doppler sample volume, wherein lies a broad range of blood flow velocities.

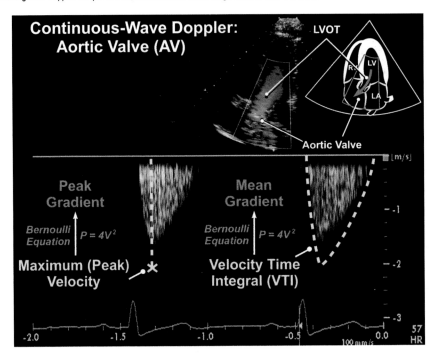

Table 4.2 OPTIMIZING THE SPECTRAL DOPPLER EXAMINATION

1. Optimize beam-vessel alignment: minimize Doppler angle (see Fig. 4.8).
2. Color flow Doppler-guided placement of Doppler sample (see Fig. 4.16).
3. Adjusting baseline and velocity scales settings (see Fig. 4.16).
4. Doppler gain settings: minimize noise and artifact.
5. Wall filter settings: minimize low frequencies (from vessel wall and valves) to optimize appearance of spectral Doppler display.
6. Sample volume size/Gate length: normally a sample volume of 2 to 5 mm is best for PW. Larger sample volumes diminish range specificity and broaden the Doppler spectrum.
7. Doppler harmonic imaging.
8. Doppler contrast imaging.

SPECTRAL DOPPLER EXAMINATION SUMMARY
Figure 4.21

Summary chart of the spectral Doppler examination. The spectral Doppler exam is an integral part of the standard transthoracic examination (see Table 5.4, Figures 4.13 and 5.4). As outlined in the standard transthoracic examination protocol, spectral Doppler is used to interrogate specific heart valves and chambers after optimizing the 2D image. The pulsed-wave (PW) and continuous-wave (CW) Doppler examination typically follow the color flow Doppler examination, which serves as a useful guide to optimal positioning of the spectral Doppler sample volume. This is especially useful when assessing abnormal flow patterns.

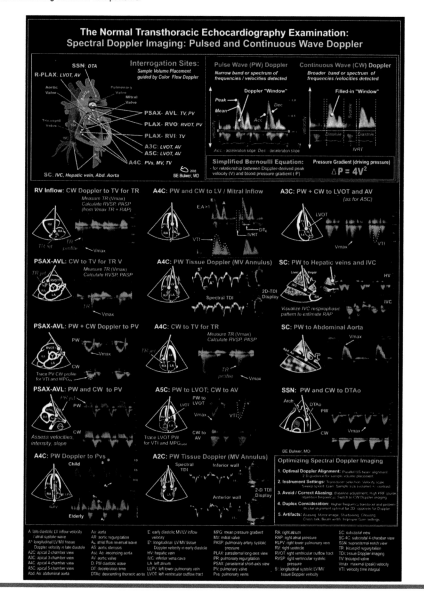

COMPARISON: CW, PW, AND COLOR FLOW DOPPLER

Table 4.3 COMPARISON OF THE MAJOR DOPPLER MODALITIES USED IN ECHOCARDIOGRAPHY

	Continuous-wave (CW) Doppler	Pulsed-wave (PW) Doppler	Color flow Doppler
Sample volume	Large (measured in cm)	Small (2-5 mm)	Large (adjustable color scan sector size)
Velocities measured	A spectrum: maximum-to-minimum (hence the term "spectral" Doppler)	A spectrum: maximum-to-minimum (hence the term "spectral" Doppler)	Mean velocity (each color pixel or voxel codes for mean velocity and flow direction on "BART" scale)
Display format	Time-velocity spectral graph	Time-velocity spectral graph	Color-coded velocity pixels (2D) and voxels (3D) superimposed on B-mode image
Spectrum of blood flow velocities detected and displayed	Wide; Spectral broadening (no "window" seen on time-velocity graphical display)	Narrow; Spectral window (but spectral broadening seen with turbulent flows)	Wide; Wide spectrum of velocities displayed as color mosaic—green color added to conventional "BART" scale
Detection of high blood flow velocities	No aliasing; accurate assessment	Aliasing; inaccurate assessment with high flow velocities	Color aliasing (even with normal intracardiac flows)
Aliasing artifact and display see Fig. 4.22	No aliasing; no Nyquist velocity limit; peak velocities on the correct side of baseline	Aliasing; Nyquist limit; aliased velocities appear on opposite side of baseline	Aliasing; color aliasing appears as color inversion on BART scale (e.g., light blue-light yellow and vice versa)
Depth resolution/ range ambiguity	Range ambiguity	Range resolution (single gate)	Range resolution (multiple gates)

2D: two-dimensional echocardiography; 3D: three-dimensional echocardiography; BART: "Blue Away Red Toward"

Figure 4.22

Comparison of hemodynamic Doppler measures. See Table 4.3.

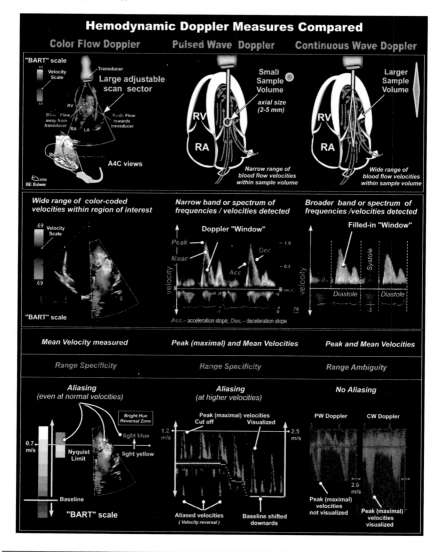

CARDIAC MECHANICS: NORMAL CARDIAC MOTION
Figure 4.23

Cardiac mechanics. Cardiac motion is complex, and it involves global translational movement as it occurs during inspiration and expiration, as well as whole heart movements during the cardiac cycle. Regionally, the heart's movements are highly orchestrated.

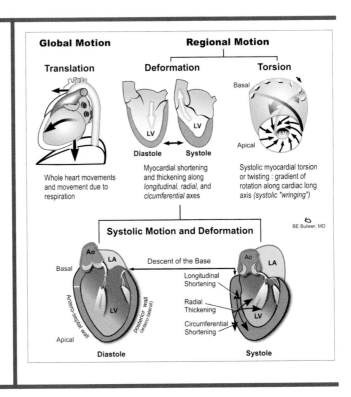

The heart does not simply "squeeze." A more accurate description is that the heart—more specifically the left ventricle—simultaneously shortens, thickens, and twists (torsion or wringing action) during systole, with reversal of these movements during diastole. The atria act in concert, exhibiting partially reciprocal movements (see Chapter 7, Figure 7.15, Left atrial dynamics).

The complex behavior of the left ventricle (LV) reflects its helical cardiac muscle fiber architecture and the elaborate innervation systems. Ventricular shortening and thickening are obvious during echocardiography. LV torsion is readily appreciated during open-heart surgery, but it is evident primarily on short-axis views of the apical LV segments.

Note: The LV endocardium and inner LV walls thicken or "squeeze" far more than the LV's outer wall. This is readily apparent on echocardiography. For this reason failure to clearly visualize the endocardium during echocardiography can lead to falsely underestimating cardiac systolic function parameters, e.g., the left ventricular ejection fraction (LVEF). See Chapter 6, Figures 6.19–6.22.

TISSUE DOPPLER IMAGING (TDI)
Figure 4.24

Tissue Doppler imaging (TDI). Longitudinal shortening and lengthening of the left ventricle (LV) can be assessed using a PW TDI technique that selectively examines the low-frequency, high-amplitude echoes arising from the myocardium instead of the high-frequency, low-amplitude echoes reflected from blood cells. *Top panel:* The TDI data can be displayed as TDI-spectral profile that shows positive systolic (S) velocities (red motion) toward the transducer plus two negative (blue motion) diastolic (E_1 and A_1) velocities that reflect biphasic LV myocardial lengthening. *Mid and bottom panel:* Alternatively, the TDI velocities can be simultaneously displayed as red tissue motion toward the transducer during systole, with blue tissue motion velocities away from the transducer during diastole.

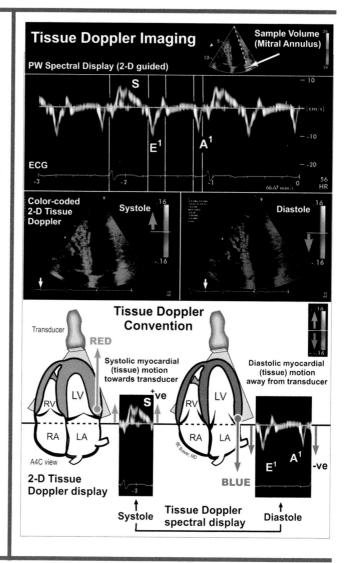

TDI-DERIVED MEASURES: VELOCITY, DISPLACEMENT, STRAIN, AND STRAIN RATE
Figure 4.25

Tissue Doppler-based parameters: 1) tissue velocity, 2) displacement (velocity × time), 3) strain (myocardial deformation), and 4) strain rate (SR) (rate of myocardial deformation). Tissue velocities merely reflect motion, but do not distinguish normal tissue motion from that of nonviable myocardial (because of tethering). Strain and strain rate measures can distinguish true contractile tissue motion from motion simply due to tethering. These measures have promising applications in patients with coronary artery disease. ε: strain; AC: aortic valve closure; ES: end systole; IVC: isovolumetric contraction; IVR: isovolumetric relaxation; MO: mitral valve opening; S: peak systolic velocity.

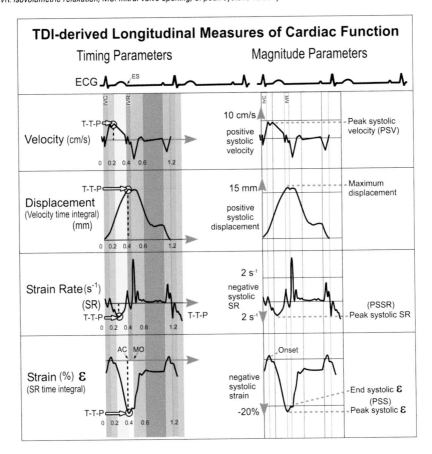

ULTRASOUND ARTIFACTS

Understanding artifacts, their mechanisms, and occurrence are important in echocardiography because: (i) they are common, (ii) their recognition is crucial for proper interpretation, and (iii) they can cause unnecessary alarm, unwarranted investigations, and inappropriate intervention.

Cardiac ultrasound artifacts may result from:

1. **Faulty equipment:** Instrument malfunction, e.g., faulty transducer, or interference, e.g., from electrocautery.
2. **Improper instrument settings:** Poor transducer selection, e.g., using a 3.5 MHz transducer with an obese patient; suboptimal imaging technique; gain settings too low or too high; inadequate dynamic range, imaging depth, scan sector width too large with color Doppler imaging.
3. **Improper or suboptimal imaging technique and/or patient characteristics:** Sonographer inexperience, "technically limited" studies in patients with obstructive lung diseases, truncal obesity, and post-chest surgery; limitations of technique, e.g., aliasing with pulsed-wave and color flow Doppler.
4. **Acoustic or songographic artifacts:** These result from interaction of ultrasound with tissues, e.g., attenuation, acoustic speckling, reverberation, mirror-image, and side lobe artifacts Figure 4.26 and Table 4.4 .

ULTRASOUND ARTIFACTS

Figure 4.26

Examples of common artifacts seen in echocardiography. Familiarity with ultrasound artifacts is crucial to optimal image acquisition and interpretation. Ultrasound artifacts are common, and are often misinterpreted. Some, like comet tail artifacts, are a minor nuisance. Others, like speckle artifacts, are useful in speckle tracking echocardiography—a recent advance based on the ubiquitous myocardial "signature" patterns that can be tracked throughout the cardiac cycle. Pulsed-wave (PW) Doppler can interrogate specific areas of flow (range specificity) but exhibits aliasing artifacts with high flow velocities seen in valvular heart disease. Color flow Doppler imaging, a PW Doppler-based technique, is also plagued by color aliasing that occurs even with normal flows (see Figure 4.22).

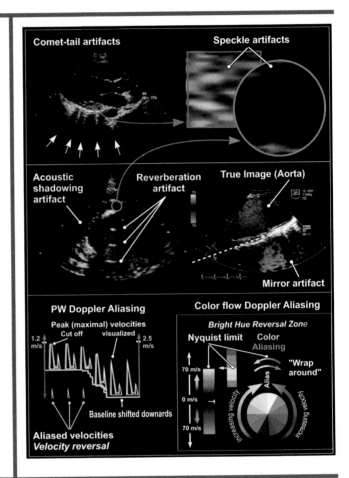

COMMON ULTRASOUND ARTIFACTS

Table 4.4 COMMON ACOUSTIC ARTIFACTS SEEN IN ECHOCARDIOGRAPHY

Acoustic artifacts	Mechanism	Examples, Comments
Attenuation artifact (acoustic shadowing) See Fig. 3.9	Progressive loss of ultrasound beam intensity and image quality with imaging distance (depth) due to reflection and scattering of the transmitted ultrasound beam. Attenuation is most marked distal to strong reflectors and manifests as image dropout or reduced image quality (acoustic shadowing). Less attenuation is seen with low-frequency transducers (1 MHz) compared to high-frequency transducers (5 MHz).	Distal to bony ribs, calcified structures, e.g., valve leaflets and annulus, prosthetic heart valves and intracardiac hardware. Air strongly reflects ultrasound. Use coupling gel on skin (to overcome the acoustic impedance difference) to aid beam transmission.
Acoustic speckling See Figs. 3.9, 3.10, and 4.26	Grainy pattern or "speckle" is normal in echocardiographic images, especially the ventricular myocardium. They result from interference patterns created by reflected ultrasound waves (echoes). They are useful in tracking cardiac motion and deformation in speckle tracking echocardiography.	Ventricular myocardium Speckles are not actual structures: constructive and destructive interference of reflected ultrasound waves (echoes) lead to this granular appearance typical of echocardiography images.
Reverberation artifact, comet tail or "ring-down" artifact See Fig. 4.26	These result from back-and-forth "ping pong" reflections (reverberations) between two highly reflective surfaces. They appear as strong linear reflections distal to the causative structure. "Comet-tail" artifacts are a type of reverberation artifact appearing distal to strong reflectors.	Ribs, pericardium, intracardiac hardware, e.g., prosthetic valves, LVAD— (left ventricular assist device) inflow. Comet-tail artifacts are almost the rule, and they are seen radiating distal to the pericardium-pleural interface.
Mirror image artifact See Fig. 4.26	An apparent duplication of a structure or Doppler signal because of strong reflector.	Aorta on transesophageal echocardiography.
Side lobe	Erroneous mapping of structures arising outside of the imaging plane (due to ultrasound beam side lobes) into the final image. Side lobe artifacts appear at the same depth as the true structures, giving rise to them.	Duplication of aortic wall within aortic lumen—may be misinterpreted as an aortic dissection flap.

(continues)

Table 4.4 COMMON ACOUSTIC ARTIFACTS SEEN IN ECHOCARDIOGRAPHY *(continued)*

Acoustic artifacts	Mechanism	Examples, Comments
Aliasing artifact See [Figs. 4.22 and 4.26]	A limitation of pulsed-wave Doppler-based techniques that erroneously displays Doppler blood velocities. Aliased PW Doppler-measured blood velocities occur when measuring high blood velocities. They appear as decapitated spectral Doppler velocities on the opposite side of the baseline. Color flow Doppler aliased velocities appear as unexpected shade of light blue, when they should instead appear as light red, or vice versa. See [Fig. 4.22].	PW Doppler measurement of aortic stenosis and mitral regurgitation. See [Figs. 6.25 and 6.29]. Adjust baseline and use continuous-wave (CW) Doppler. Color flow Doppler mapping of high blood flow velocities; mosaic colors indicating the turbulent flows seen. Note: color flow aliasing is also commonly seen with normal intracardiac flow velocities.

The Transthoracic Echocardiography Examination

PART 2

CHAPTER 5

Orientation, Maneuvers, and the Examination Protocol

TRANSDUCER SCAN PLANE, INDEX MARK, AND SCAN SECTOR IMAGE DISPLAY

The geometric ultrasound beam or sector scan is generated by rapid sweeps of the ultrasound beam (of the phased array transducer) through the region of interest or anatomical scan plane as illustrated earlier in Figures 3.6, 3.11, and 3.12 . Conceptually, the ultrasound beam, therefore, is a pie-shaped beam, as shown in Figure 5.1a . Note the position of the index mark—a guide to transducer beam orientation during the examination. The index mark may be a palpable ridge or a depression, with or without light to aid transducer orientation in a dimly lit room. By convention, the index mark indicates the part of the image plane that appears on the right side of the image display Figure 5.1b .

Figure 5.1a

Transducer scan plane and index mark.

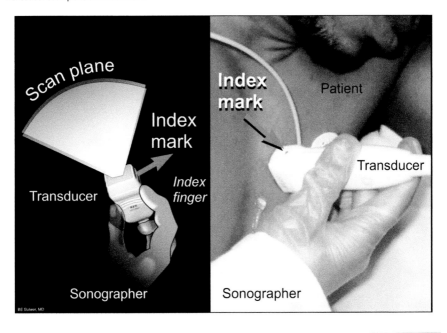

Figure 5.1b

The concept of the index mark, the transducer scan plane, and corresponding image display using the apical 4-chamber view.

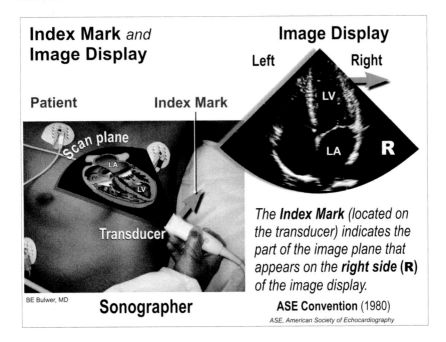

Index Mark *and* Image Display

Image Display

Patient   Index Mark   Left   Right

Scan plane

LV

LA

LA   **R**

Transducer

BE Bulwer, MD

Sonographer

*The **Index Mark** (located on the transducer) indicates the part of the image plane that appears on the **right side** (**R**) of the image display.*

ASE Convention (1980)

ASE, American Society of Echocardiography

Figure 5.2

Transducer position, index mark, anatomically correct image orientation with the scan plane, and the corresponding image display. Note the position of the index mark (red arrow) at each stage. Most echocardiographic laboratories use the apex up projection for the apical four-chamber display. Compare with Figures 7.4–7.6.

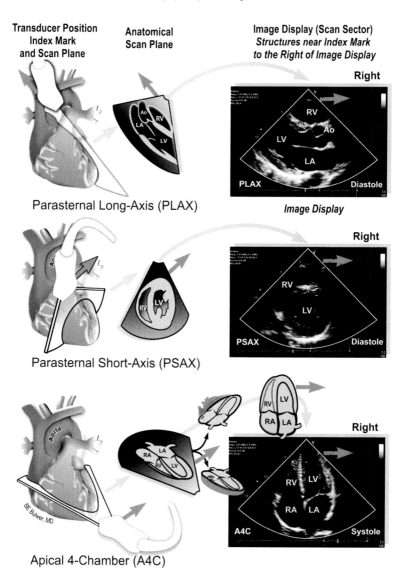

Transducer Position Index Mark and Scan Plane

Anatomical Scan Plane

Image Display (Scan Sector) *Structures near Index Mark to the Right of Image Display*

Parasternal Long-Axis (PLAX)

Image Display

Parasternal Short-Axis (PSAX)

Apical 4-Chamber (A4C)

TRANSDUCER MANEUVERS

Four major transducer movements within each transducer position (windows) are described—sliding, angling, rotating, and tilting [Figure 5.3]. The aim of these maneuvers is to optimally acquire images of the region of interest. Transducer movements are fluid and often subtle. A sound knowledge of 3D echocardiographic anatomy is a prequisite for efficient maneuvering and identification of important cardiac structures during the examination.

Figure 5.3

Transducer maneuvers: angling, rotation, and tilting. See Figure 6.58 for description of the recommended sliding maneuvers when acquiring the parasternal short axis (PSAX) views.

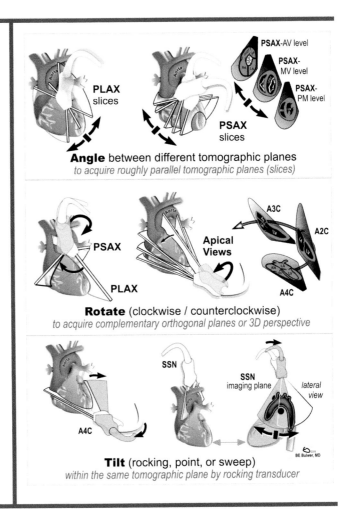

Angle between different tomographic planes
to acquire roughly parallel tomographic planes (slices)

Rotate (clockwise / counterclockwise)
to acquire complementary orthogonal planes or 3D perspective

Tilt (rocking, point, or sweep)
within the same tomographic plane by rocking transducer

CHECKLIST: THE TRANSTHORACIC EXAMINATION

Table 5.1 TTE EXAMINATION CHECKLISTS

TTE Examination Checklists

Equipment Checklist

• **Pre-Scanning**

Ergonomics
Sonographer preference (left/right side)
Machine settings, Presets
    Transducer (MHz) selection
    Gain settings
    Harmonic imaging
    ECG signal
Warm transducer coupling gel

• **During the Examination**

Note index mark for correct image
    orientation
Firm, but gentle pressure (Do not hurt!)
Appropriate windows and transducer
    maneuvers. Movements often subtle
Optimal image aquisiton: be not hostage
    to a "fixed" transducer position:
    Go wherever you get the best image.
Optimize region of interest:
Apply appropriate modality: e.g. 2D, M-Mode
    Color, PW, CW, Tissue Doppler, 3D
Optimize 2D controls: *automatic / manual*
    e.g. Depth, Sector width, (frame rate)
    Gain, Compress, Dynamic range,
    Gain settings
Optimize Doppler controls: CW, PW, Color
    Optimal alignment, Velocity Range, Wall
    filters, Sample volume, Avoid aliasing
    Color scan sector width, Color gain,
    Color velocity scale/PRF
Acquire images and video loops
Measurements and quantitative parameters

• **Post Scanning**

End study
Documentation
Transmit images
Equipment care, storage, maintenance

BE Bulwer, MD

Patient Checklist

• **Pre-Scanning**

Patient instruction and reassurance re:
    exam procedure, expectations, *etc.*
Patient entry menu
History and Indications for the exam
ECG leads
Transducer (coupling) gel (keep warm)
Weight
Blood pressure (*esp.* for Doppler exam)
Partial undress (modesty)
Optimal patient position (patient comfort)

• **During the Examination**

Interactive examination
Optimal patient comfort
Patient modesty
Appropriate communication of findings
    with patient

• **Post Scanning**

Remove ECG leads, transducer gel, dress
Patient handover
Enter examination findings
Appropriate communication of findings
Safe patient handover or Discharge

Patient
Communication, Comfort,
Modesty
Safety
Individual characteristics
Medical, surgical status

Equipment
Optimal instrument
settings
Warm coupling gel
ECG leads
BP monitor

Sonographer
Knowlegde
Training
Experience

Before you begin, note the checklists in [Table 5.1]. Most sonographers prefer a dimly lit room to improve the image contrast. Patient comfort and safety are paramount. Apply ECG leads before commencement of the examination.

PATIENT CHARACTERISTICS AND EXAMINATION CAVEATS

Table 5.2 PATIENT CHARACTERISTICS AND EXAMINATION CAVEATS

Individual patient characteristics	Examination caveats
Normal individual variation	The recommended transducer positions or "windows" are a good guide only. Don't be held hostage by the recommended protocol. Acquire views using the best windows.
Normal patient with "difficult windows"	Consider repositioning patient, including use of the steep left lateral decubitus or semi-Fowler (partially sitting up) positions.
Body habitus, including obesity; pregnancy	Obese patients pose a challenge on many fronts. Low-frequency transducers (less than 2.5 MHz) are necessary ± ultrasound contrast agents. Women in the third trimester should be examined in the left lateral decubitus position, as supine position may lead to compromised vascular flow.
The anxious but otherwise normal patient	Reassurance. Provide measured information about study results. Leave the official interpretation to the attending physician or care provider.
Age: infants, children	Children are a special challenge, often requiring special equipment ± sedation. With premature and newborn infants, or older infants with cartilaginous chest walls, use a 7.5 MHz and 5 MHz transducer, respectively.
Dextrocardia	Suspect when you can't see normal windows when no information is available from the history. Palpate apex beat.
Chest wall pathology, e.g., scoliosis, pectus excavatum	Use the windows that provide the best views.
Lung disease, e.g., emphysema, pneumothorax	Hyperinflated lung fields usually result in low parasternal windows—almost near the "apical" area. Subcostal windows are often the best.
Post chest surgery	The subcostal examination may be the only "free" window. Consider transesophageal echocardiography (TEE) or other cardiac imaging modality as necessary.
Patient in the intensive care units/critical care units; very ill or distressed patients	Perform a targeted or focused echo examination ± TEE; Doppler hemodynamic studies are often important.
Emergency room patients, e.g., chest trauma, chest pain, cardiac arrest	Perform a targeted or focused echo examination.

TIPS FOR OPTIMIZING IMAGE ACQUISITION FOR 2D MEASUREMENTS

Table 5.3 TIPS FOR OPTIMAL IMAGE ACQUISITION

Aim	Methods and techniques
Minimize translational motion	Quiet or suspended respiration (at end-expiration)
Maximize image resolution	Image at minimum depth necessary Highest possible transducer frequency Adjust gains, dynamic range, transmit and lateral gain controls appropriately Frame rate $\geq$ 30/sec Harmonic imaging B-color imaging (to optimize image contrast)
Avoid apical foreshortening	Steep lateral decubitus position Cut-out mattress Do not rely on the palpable apical impulse
Maximize endocardial border delineation	Use harmonic imaging and/or contrast agents to enhance delineation of endocardial borders
Identify end-diastole and end-systole	Use mitral valve motion and ventricular cavity size rather than reliance on ECG

THE EXAMINATION PROTOCOL

The comprehensive transthoracic echocardiography examination begins at the left parasternal window, followed by the apical, subcostal, and suprasternal windows (Table 5.4), (Figures 5.4–5.6).

Each standard echocardographic view (Figure 5.4) is defined by the:

- **Transducer position (window):** e.g., parasternal (P), apical (A), subcostal (SC), and suprasternal notch (SSN)
- **Echocardiographic imaging plane:** e.g., long-axis (LAX), short-axis (SAX), or four-chamber (4C)
- **Cardiac structures or regions of interest:** e.g., left ventricular inflow-outflow, right ventricular inflow, or aortic valve level

At each window, the normal examination protocol (Table 5.4) is to perform:

- **2D examination:** (Figure 5.4) Optimize and acquire each view. Obtain linear and volumetric measures where applicable. Assess normal and abnormal cardiac structure and function as the examination proceeds. Confirm findings in subsequent views as the examination proceeds.
- **M-mode examination:** Use this modality to time cardiac events and structures of interest. Perform linear and derived measurements where applicable (Figures 6.12–6.14).
- **Color flow Doppler examination:** Visualize "angiographic" blood flow velocities and flow patterns within cardiac chambers, the great vessels, and across heart valves (Figure 4.13).
- **Spectral pulsed wave (PW) and continuous-wave (CW) Doppler examination:** Quantify blood flow velocities within cardiac chambers, the great vessels, and across heart valves (Figure 4.21).
- **Tissue Doppler imaging (TDI):** PW TDI to the mitral annulus to quantify myocardial tissue velocities at specific regions (Figures 4.24, 7.22, 7.23).
- **3D imaging:** (Figures 6.11, 6.65, 7.12) 3D is particularly useful in quantification of the left ventricle, e.g., LV mass and volumes (Figures 6.11, 6.65, 7.12).
- **Ultrasound contrast agents:** Use where indicated, e.g., to improve endocardial border delineation.

EXAMINATION PROTOCOL: 2D TRANSTHORACIC ECHOCARDIOGRAPHY

Table 5.4 TWO-DIMENSIONAL (2D) AND DOPPLER TTE EXAM PROTOCOL

Two-Dimensional (2D) and Doppler TTE*Exam Protocol

1. **PARASTERNAL LONG-AXIS (PLAX)** - Depth 20-24 cm on **2D**; Optimize & Acquire
2. **PARASTERNAL LONG-AXIS (PLAX)** - Depth 15-16 cm on **2D**; Optimize & Acquire
   a. **M-mode** - Sweep through *MV/AV, Aortic Root, LA, LV*
   b. Measure *Aortic root* (*end systole* on **2-D** or **M-mode**)
   c. Suspected Aortic stenosis (AS) measure *LVOT* 1 cm below leaflets (end systole; **2D**)
   d. Measure *LA* (*end-diastole*; **2-D** or **M-mode**)
   e. Measure *IVS end-diastole / LV internal diameter/Posterior wall thickness* (**2D or M-mode**)
   f. Measure *LV internal diameter* end-systole (**2-D or M-mode**)
   g. Zoom on *MV/AV*
   h. **Color Doppler** on *MV/AV* for mitral (MR) or aortic regurgitation (AR)
3. **RV INFLOW** - Depth 20 cm, then 15-16 cm (**2D**); Optimize & Acquire
   a. Zoom on *TV*
   b. **Color Doppler** -*TV* for TR
   c. **CW Doppler** -*TV* for TR for maximal velocity; (**RV OUTFLOW** optional)
4. **PARASTERNAL SHORT-AXIS (PSAX)** on **2D**; Optimize & Acquire
   a. **2D** *AV level*; zoom on *AV*, **Color Doppler** for AR width
   b. **Color Doppler** *TV* for TR, **CW Doppler** TR for velocity
   c. **Color Doppler** *PV* for PR, **PW and CW Doppler**
   d. **2D** image of *PA Bifurcation*, **PW Doppler** *from RVOT to Bifurcation* (look for PDA)
   e. **2D** *MV level* (**Color Doppler** optional)
   f. **2D** *LV-Papillary Muscle level*
   g. **2D** *LV-Apical level*
5. **APICAL 4-CHAMBER (A4C)** - Depth 20-24 cm on **2D**; Optimize and Acquire
6. **APICAL 4-CHAMBER (A4C)** - Depth 15-16 cm; Optimize & Acquire
   a. Decrease depth to visualize *LV Apex*
   b. **Color Doppler** *MV* for MR
   c. **PW Doppler** *Pulmonary Veins*
   d. **PW Doppler** *Mitral Inflow (Tips of MV leaflets in LV)* for velocity, E/A ratio
   e. **CW Doppler** *MV*
   f. **PW Tissue Doppler** at level of *Mitral Annulus* (lateral and septal), scale 20:20
   g. Visualize *RV*, **Color Doppler** to TV
   h. **CW Doppler** if TR present
7. **APICAL 5-CHAMBER (A5C)** on **2D**; Optimize & Acquire
   a. Visualize *AV*
   b. **Color Doppler** *AV* for AR
   c. **PW Doppler** along *LV Septum from Apex towards AV*
   d. If AS: **PW Doppler** 1cm below AV; freeze and trace VTI-1
   e. If AS: **CW Doppler** through AV; freeze and trace for VT1-2 (if Afib. trace 5 beats in a row
8. **APICAL 2-CHAMBER (A2C)** on **2D**; Optimize & Acquire
   a. **Color Doppler** for MR; **PW Tissue Doppler** to *Mitral Annulus* (anterior, inferior) optional
9. **APICAL 3-CHAMBER (A3C): APICAL LONG-AXIS (ALAX)** on **2D**; Optimize
   a. **Color Doppler** *MV/AV* for MR and AR
10. **SUBCOSTAL 4-CHAMBER (SC-4C)** on **2D**; Optimize & Acquire
    a. **Color Doppler** *Atrial Septum* for ASD
    b. **Color Doppler** *RV* for TR
    c. Visualize *IVC*; **Color Doppler**, Measure *IVC*, and **PW Doppler** *hepatic veins*
11. **SUPRASTERNAL NOTCH (SSN)** - Depth ~24 cm, on **2D**; Optimize & Acquire
    a. **Color Doppler** and **PW Doppler** to *Descending Thoracic Aorta*

*TTE: Transthoracic Echocardiography (Comprehensive Adult Protocol)

Figure 5.4

A panoramic depiction of the 2D transthoracic examination, beginning with the PLAX view, and showing the standard transducer positions ("windows"), imaging planes, and views. See corresponding protocol outlined in Table 5.4 and Figure 5.6, along with the corresponding color flow Doppler and spectral Doppler examination (Figures 4.13 and 4.21).

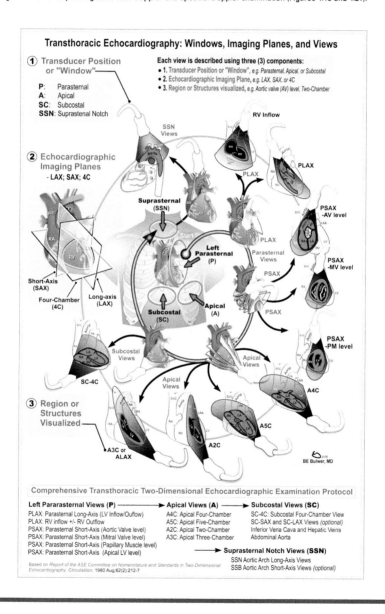

Transthoracic Echocardiography: Windows, Imaging Planes, and Views

(1) Transducer Position or "Window"

Each view is described using three (3) components:
- 1. Transducer Position or "Window", e.g. Parasternal, Apical, or Subcostal
- 2. Echocardiographic Imaging Plane, e.g. LAX, SAX, or 4C
- 3. Region or Structures visualized, e.g. Aortic valve (AV) level, Two-Chamber

P: Parasternal
A: Apical
SC: Subcostal
SSN: Suprastenal Notch

(2) Echocardiographic Imaging Planes
- LAX; SAX; 4C

Short-Axis (SAX)

Four-Chamber (4C) Long-axis (LAX)

(3) Region or Structures Visualized

SSN Views

Suprasternal (SSN)

Start

Left Parasternal (P)

Subcostal (SC)

Apical (A)

RV Inflow

PLAX

PLAX

Parasternal Views

PSAX

PSAX -AV level

PSAX -MV level

PSAX

PSAX -PM level

Subcostal Views

Apical Views

A4C

A5C

SC-4C

Apical Views

A2C

A3C or ALAX

BE Bulwer, MD

Comprehensive Transthoracic Two-Dimensional Echocardiographic Examination Protocol

Left Pararasternal Views (P) ──▶ **Apical Views (A)** ──▶ **Subcostal Views (SC)**

PLAX: Parasternal Long-Axis (LV Inflow/Ouflow)
PLAX: RV inflow +/- RV Outflow
PSAX: Parasternal Short-Axis (Aortic Valve level)
PSAX: Parasternal Short-Axis (Mitral Valve level)
PSAX: Parasternal Short-Axis (Papillary Muscle level)
PSAX: Parasternal Short-Axis (Apical LV level)

A4C: Apical Four-Chamber
A5C: Apical Five-Chamber
A2C: Apical Two-Chamber
A3C: Apical Three-Chamber

SC-4C: Subcostal Four-Chamber View
SC-SAX and SC-LAX Views (optional)
Inferior Vena Cava and Hepatic Veins
Abdominal Aorta

──▶ **Suprasternal Notch Views (SSN)**

SSN Aortic Arch Long-Axis Views
SSB Aortic Arch Short-Axis Views (optional)

Based on Report of the ASE Committee on Nomenclature and Standards in Two-Dimensional Echocardiography. Circulation. 1980 Aug;62(2):212-7

Figure 5.5

The standard transducer windows.

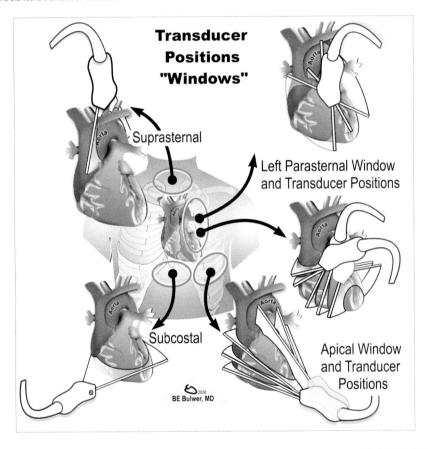

The normal sequence of the adult transthoracic examination is as follows
Figure 5.4 :

1. **Left Parasternal Views:** Parasternal long-axis (PLAX); right ventricular (RV) inflow ± RV outflow; parasternal short-axis (PSAX) views
2. **Apical Views:** Apical 4-chamber (A4C); apical 2-chamber (A2C); apical long-axis (ALAX) or apical 3-chamber (A3C) views
3. **Subcostal Views:** Subcostal 4-chamber (SC-4C); inferior vena cava (IVC); abdominal aorta (Abd. A) views
4. **Suprasternal Notch Views (SSN):** Suprasternal long-axis view of the aortic arch

Figure 5.6

Tabular depiction of echocardiographic windows, imaging planes, views (scan plane anatomy), and the major structures or regions visualized.

Transducer Position "Window"	Imaging Plane	Views	Region or Structures Visualized
Parasternal (left)	**Long-Axis (PLAX)**	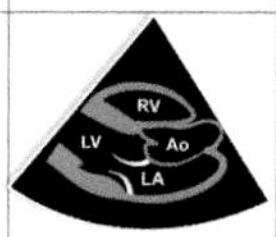	LV inflow-outflow: LA-LV-Ao. RV inflow: RA, RV *RV outflow: RVOT, PA
Parasternal (left)	**Short-Axis (PSAX)**	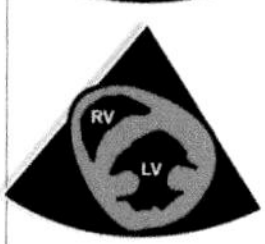	Aortic valve (AV) level Pulmonary bifurcation Mitral valve (MV) level Papillary muscle level Apical level
Apical	**4-Chamber (A4C - A5C)**	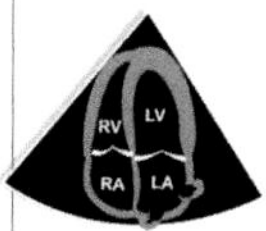	A4C: LA, LV, RA, RV A4C + Coronary sinus A4C + Aortic root = A5C
Apical **Apical**	**Long-Axis (A3C)** **2-Chamber (A2C)**	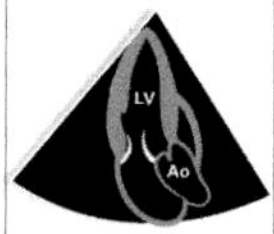	A3C: LA, LV, Aortic root (LV inflow-outflow) A2C: LA, LV
Subcostal	**4-Chamber (SC-4C)**	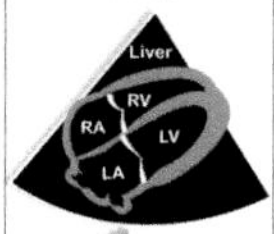	SC-4C: LA, LV, RA, RV *"Sweep" from horizontal to frontal planes
Subcostal	**Short-Axis* (SC-SAX)**	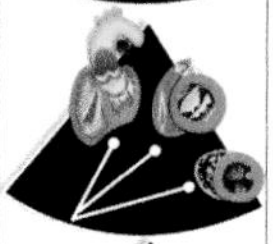	*SC-SAX "Sweep" apex to base - plane like PSAX views
Subcostal	**Long-Axis Short-Axis* (IVC, Aorta)**	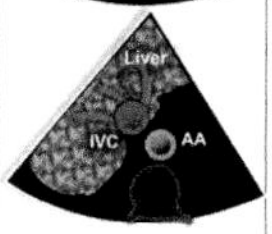	IVC: inferior vena cava AA: abdominal aorta Hepatic veins +/- viscera
Suprasternal Notch	**Long-Axis Short-Axis* (SSN)**	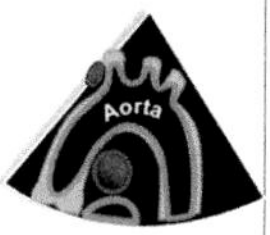	SSN - Aortic arch LAX *SSN - Aortic arch SAX

*Optional: when indicated

BE Bulwer. MD

CHAPTER 6

Left Parasternal Views

Figure 6.1

Left parasternal window, transducer scan planes, and views. From the left parasternal position, a family of long-axis and short-axis views are obtained by sweeping (or angling) the transducer along the cardiac long axis and short axis as shown.

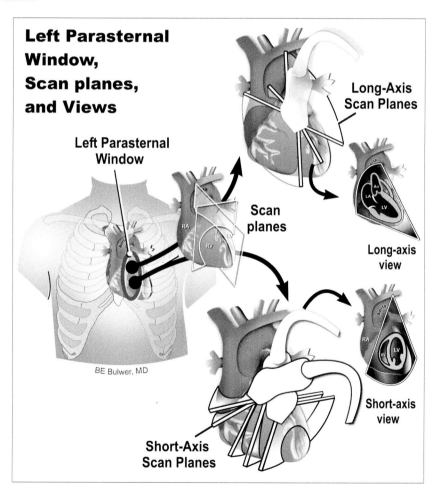

Left Parasternal Window, Scan planes, and Views

Left Parasternal Window

Scan planes

Long-Axis Scan Planes

Long-axis view

Short-Axis Scan Planes

Short-axis view

BE Bulwer, MD

The following standard parasternal views are obtained.

1. Parasternal long-axis (PLAX) view of the left ventricular (LV) inflow and outflow tracts Figures 6.2–6.5.
2. Parasternal long-axis (PLAX) view of the right ventricular (RV) inflow tract, hereafter called the RV inflow view Figures 6.2–6.5.
3. Parasternal long-axis (PLAX) of the right ventricular (RV) outflow tract, hereafter called the RV outflow view Figures 6.2–6.4.
4. The parasternal short-axis (PSAX) views—at multiple short-axis levels Figures 6.49, 6.50, beginning with the PSAX view at the level of the aortic valve (PSAX-AVL), at the level of the pulmonary artery bifurcation (PSAX-PAB), the level of the mitral valve (PSAX-MVL); the mid-LV level or papillary muscle level (PSAX-PML), and at the level of the LV apical segments (PSAX-apical level), including the apical cap of the LV.

LEFT PARASTERNAL VIEWS

Under normal circumstances, the left parasternal window is where the adult examination begins. Sweeping (or sequential angulations of) the transducer through the cardiac long-axis and short-axis planes produces an unlimited family of views. However, for practical reasons, only a standard selection of representative and reproducible views are recorded `Figures 5.4, 6.1, 6.4, and 6.50`.

The parasternal long-axis (PLAX) view is one of the most important views. It provides the initial impression of overall cardiac structure and function, especially of left-sided cardiac structures `Figures 6.2–6.5`. It marks the start of the adult transthoracic examination. Its orientation perpendicular to the ultrasound beam delivers optimal B-mode images, and is especially useful for definition of the LV endocardium. Endocardial border definition is a prerequisite for obtaining accurate linear and volumetric measures, which are clinically useful parameters of LV function. The RV inflow and outflow views, as their names indicate, are used to assess right-sided cardiac chamber structure and function, including assessment of RV inflow via the tricuspid valve and outflow via the pulmonary valves `Figures 6.2–6.4`. The parasternal short-axis (PSAX) views are obtained at multiple levels parallel to the LV short-axis plane `Figures 6.49, 6.50`. They are acquired sequentially, beginning at the level of the aortic valve (PSAX-AVL); at the level of the pulmonary artery bifurcation (PSAX-PAB); at the level of the mitral valve (PSAX-MVL); at the mid-LV level or papillary muscle level (PSAX-PML); and at the level of the LV apical segments (PSAX-apical level), including the apical cap of the LV.

Patient and transducer positioning

Patient comfort and safety are paramount and should adhere to best practice guidelines. Patient comfort is a particular challenge throughout an examination that may average 30 to 45 minutes, including the need to shift positions and the need to acquire images—especially the apical and subcostal views—during short periods of breath-holding in end-expiration.

Anteriorly, most of the heart is covered by the bony rib cage and the lungs; these are both obstacles to ultrasound imaging. The raison d'être for the left parasternal window is the presence of the sonographically strategic cardiac notch—the lung-free space created by an absent middle lobe of the left lung `Figures 2.4, 2.11, 2.12`. This space extends just 2 to 3 cm to the left of the sternal border, and it overlies the pericardium covering the right ventricle. The welcomed presence of the cardiac notch, however, is frustrated by the presence of the intervening ribs (costal cartilages) that reduce the size of the left parasternal window. Positioning the patient in left lateral decubitus position, however, normally increases the size of the left parasternal window. This is due to the effect of gravity on the lung—causing it to fall away from the midline—as well as the movement of the heart (including the apex) closer to the chest wall.

Transducer maneuvers

Gently but firmly apply the transducer probe (with warm ultrasound coupling gel to create an airless seal) to the left parasternal window in the 2nd to the 5th inter-costal space, and as close as possible to the left sternal border Figure 6.1 . The palpable sternal notch marks the level where the 2nd costal cartilage articulates with the manubrosternal junction. Below this lies the 2nd intercostal space Figures 2.2, 2.11, 2.12 , Table 2.1 . The subsequent intercostal spaces can therefore be palpably indentified using this landmark.

When oriented parallel to the long-axis plane of the heart (for the parasternal long-axis views), the transducer scan plane is oriented along a line extending from the right shoulder to the left loin, with the transducer index mark directed toward the 10 o'clock position Figures 6.2–6.8 .

LEFT PARASTERNAL LONG-AXIS SCAN PLANES AND VIEWS
Figure 6.2

The family of parasternal long-axis (PLAX) scan planes. **Scan plane 1:** PLAX scan plane through the long axis of the left ventricle (LV), known simply as the PLAX scan plane. **Scan plane 2:** PLAX scan plane angled through the right atrium (RA) and right ventricle (RV) and commonly called the RV inflow scan plane. **Scan plane 3:** PLAX scan plane through the right ventricular outflow-main pulmonary artery, known as the RV outflow scan plane. Note that these scan planes are not fixed, and the optimal alignment should be adjusted to visualize the desired anatomical structures or region of interest.

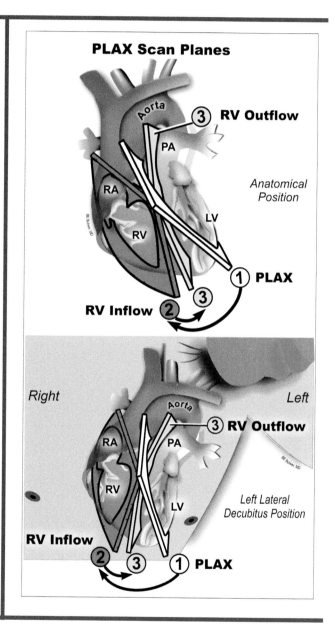

Figure 6.3

PLAX family or sweep of scan planes with patient in the left lateral decubitus position. Note the approximate landmarks and transducer maneuvers.

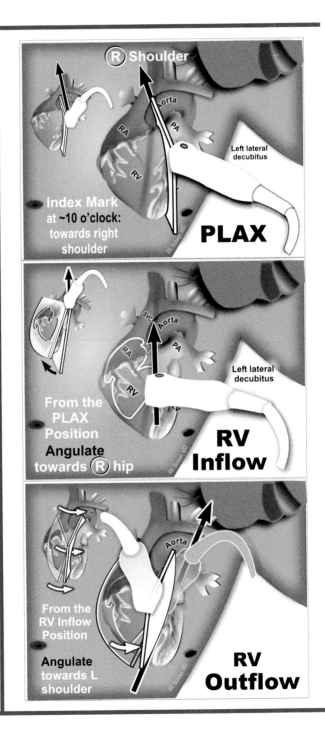

Figure 6.4

Parasternal long-axis family of scan planes, scan plane anatomy, and scan sector image displays. Note the cross-sectional anatomy and the corresponding image displays that result when the scan plane sweeps from right (RV inflow view) to left (RV outflow view).

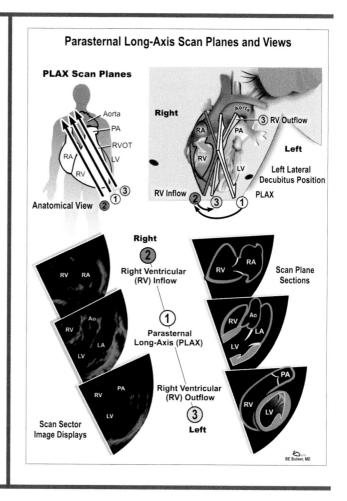

The PLAX view is where the adult transthoracic examination begins (label 1). This is because the primarily landmark cardiac structures—the right ventricle (RV), left ventricle (LV), aortic root (Ao), and left atrium (LA), and the mitral and aortic valves—can be readily aligned along the cardiac long axis in the PLAX view Figures 6.2, 6.3 . This serves as a navigational reference plane from which subsequent parasternal views are sought. Angling the transducer toward the right hip brings into view the RV inflow view (label 2). Angling toward the left shoulder brings into view the RV outflow plane (label 3).

Figure 6.5

Anatomical scan planes and image displays of parasternal long-axis (PLAX) view (A) and right ventricular (RV) inflow view (B). In the anatomical views (left panel), note the transducer scan plane, the scan plane anatomy, and the position of the transducer index mark (red arrow) when angling or sweeping the scan plane from A to B. When viewed from the left lateral perspective (right panel)—like opening the pages of a book (not exactly a mirror image)—note how the scan plane anatomy corresponds with the scan sector image displays.

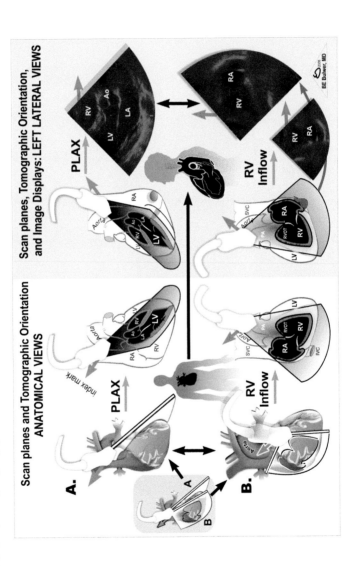

LEFT PARASTERNAL LONG-AXIS (PLAX) VIEW

Patient and transducer positioning

With the patient in the left lateral position, place the transducer in 3rd or 4th left intercostal space (LICS) with the index mark pointing toward the left shoulder, or approximately in the 10 o'clock position Figures 6.6a, 6.6b .

Transducer maneuvers

Apply generous amounts of transducer coupling gel to the transducer face, and quickly scan along the left parasternal border to get a quick impression of which intercostal space (2nd–5th) or patient position will deliver the best views. The recommended starting point is just a guide, so don't be held hostage to it. Use whatever intercostal space or patient position that delivers the best PLAX views Figures 6.6–6.9 .

Transducer scan plane orientation and anatomy

Note scan plane orientation with patient in the anatomical and left lateral positions Figures 6.2–6.5, 6.7–6.9 .

2D scan sector image display

Scan at depths of 20–24 cm to visualize cardiac and extracardiac structures, e.g., descending thoracic aorta or possible pleural effusion. Identify, optimize, and record images by adjusting gain settings, depth, and sector width accordingly. Decrease depth to 15–16 cm for closer views of cardiac structures or other regions of interest. Record images at each step Figures 6.8, 6.9 . Perform the required measurements Figure 6.15 . Assess cardiac structure and function as the examination proceeds, and confirm normal and abnormal findings using subsequent views Table 6.1 .

M-Mode Examination

M-mode examination of the PLAX view provides important data about the aortic and mitral valves, as well as linear dimensions of cardiac chambers. Perform M-mode sweeps through the aortic valve, mitral valve, and the left ventricle just distal to the tips of the mitral leaflets. Perform the required measurement Figures 6.12–6.14 .

Color flow Doppler exam

Optimize control settings, and interrogate the aortic and mitral valves Figures 6.16, 6,17 for possible aortic and mitral pathology Table 6.1 and Figures 6.24–6.29 .

PW Doppler exam

This is generally not performed on the PLAX view because of nonparallel alignment with normal cardiac chambers. However, if a ventricular septal defect Figure 6.34 of the membranous or trabecular septum is seen on the color Doppler exam, interrogate using PW and CW Doppler.

CW Doppler exam

This is generally not performed on the PLAX view (as for PW Doppler).

Coronary artery segments visualized on the PLAX view

Correlate abnormalities of ventricular wall motion and thickening with their corresponding coronary artery supply. Corroborate findings on subsequent views Figure 6.10 .

Findings and Summaries

Assess cardiac structure and function as the examination proceeds. Use a systematic approach. Confirm normal and abnormal findings using subsequent views Table 6.1 , Figures 6.18–6.34 .

PLAX VIEW: PATIENT POSITIONING, TRANSDUCER PLACEMENT, AND SCAN PLANE
Figure 6.6a

Patient and transducer positioning: parasternal long-axis view (PLAX).

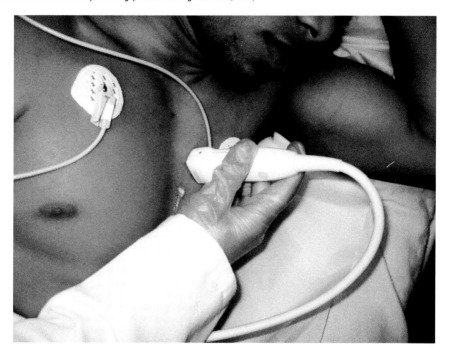

Place the transducer (after application of ultrasound coupling gel) to the left parasternal window, just lateral to the sternum. The palpable sternal notch corresponds to the 2nd intercostal space (Figures 2.2, 2.4 ; compare Figures 2.11, 2.12 ; see Table 2.1). Note transducer index mark pointing toward the 10 o'clock position (head and neck at the 12 o'clock position).

Figure 6.6b

Patient and transducer position: parasternal long-axis views (PLAX).

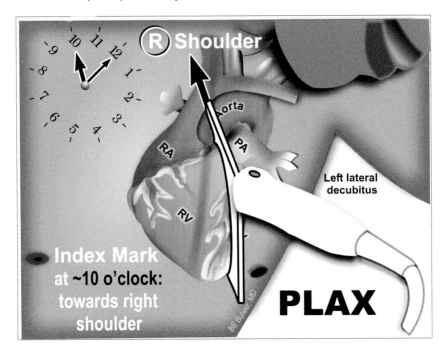

Note the position of the index mark. The scan plane is oriented along a line connecting the right shoulder to the left flank. However, do not be hostage to these parameters. Many factors affect cardiac topography and position Table 2.2 .

PLAX VIEW: SCAN PLANE, ANATOMY, AND SCAN SECTOR DISPLAY
Figure 6.7

Panoramic perspectives of the parasternal long-axis (PLAX) scan plane, scan plane anatomy, and image display.

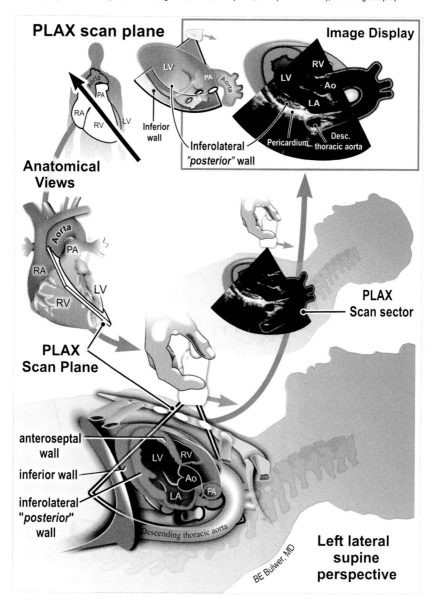

When properly acquired, the PLAX scan plane transects the major cardiac structures shown. It is the inferolateral wall (using the current nomenclature for naming cardiac walls), and not the inferior or diaphragmatic wall, through which the PLAX scan plane exits. The traditional nomenclature, "posterior" wall, is still widely used. Some authorities maintain that the PLAX view should ideally scan that area of the inferolateral wall between the papillary muscles (without recording either muscle), which are located at ~4 o'clock and ~8 o'clock positions on short-axis views Figures 2.6, 2.7, 6.62–6.63 . This is where the left ventricular (LV) diameter is maximal, and the scan plane parallel to the true long axis of the LV.

PLAX VIEW: SCAN SECTOR ANATOMY
Figure 6.8

Parasternal long-axis (PLAX) scan plane. *Ao: ascending aorta; DTAo: descending thoracic aorta; LA: left atrium; LV: left ventricle; RV: right ventricle.*

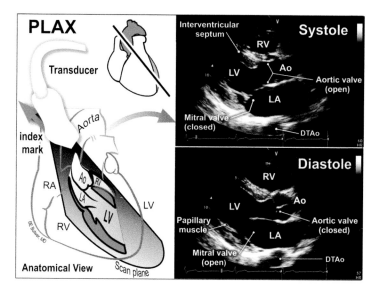

Figure 6.9

PLAX scan sector image display and cross-sectional anatomy (see Figure 2.6). Assess global measures of LV function, including LV ejection fraction (Figures 6.18–6.20). Assess normal and abnormal structure and function, and correlate on subsequent views (Table 6.1, Figures 6.24–6.34).

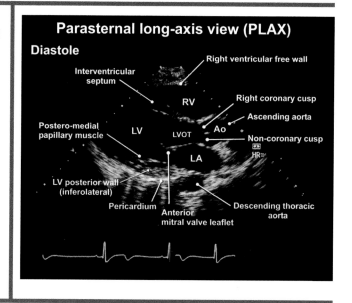

Figure 6.10

The parasternal long-axis (PLAX) view and corresponding coronary artery territories and LV segments.

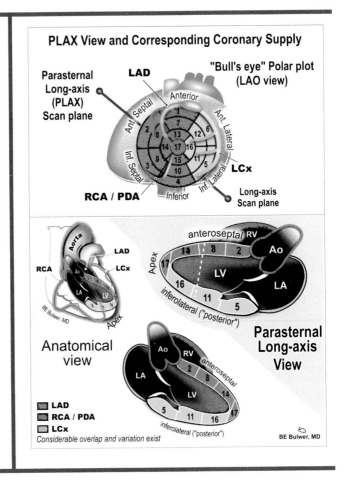

Coronary artery disease is the most common cause of regional ventricular wall motion abnormalities, which manifest variously as hypokinetic, akinetic, dyskinetic, or aneurysmal wall segments, along with impaired systolic thickening of the ventricular walls Figures 2.9, 6.21–6.23 . Note that the endocardium thickens to a much greater degree than the endocardium (see Wall Scoring, Figures 6.21, 6.22).

Therefore, during the transthoracic examination, correlate such findings as the examination proceeds. Compare with Figures 2.9, 6.23, 6.65, 7.13, 7.36, 7.42 .

PLAX VIEW: 3D PERSPECTIVES
Figure 6.11

Such real-time 3D (RT3D) data can be rapidly acquired for assessment cardiac structure and function. Full-volume echocardiography is especially useful for assessment of left ventricular function indices, e.g., ventricular mass, volumes, ejection fraction, and (dys)synchrony (see Figures 2.6, 2.7, 6.64, 7.12).

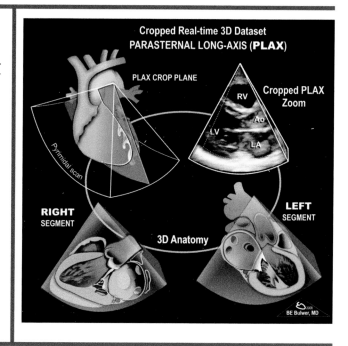

During the complete three-dimensional (3D) echocardiography examination, the protocol involves acquiring a pyramidal full-volume data set from the standard echocardiographic windows: parasternal, apical, and subcostal (optional). Additionally, color Doppler interrogation of the cardiac valves, atrial and ventricular septa, and the descending thoracic aorta is executed using the four standard windows.

The acquired pyramidal full volume can be bisected or cropped along the standard echocardiographic planes, or along the heart's coronal, sagittal, and transverse planes. Proprietary software is used for multiple off-line analyses of ventricular structure and function, akin to parameters used during the standard 2D examination.

PLAX VIEW: M-MODE EXAMINATION OF THE AORTIC VALVE AND MEASUREMENTS
Figure 6.12

Normal M-mode examination of the parasternal long-axis (PLAX) view at the level of the aortic valve. *Top panel.* Panoramic perspective of the M-mode display—a one-dimensional "ice-pick" "view of image" depth over time. The M-mode cursor (dashed line) is aligned perpendicular to the aortic root (Ao) and passes through the structures shown. Note the normal anterior movement of the aortic root during systole and the cyclical changes in left atrial (LA) dimensions. The right and left aortic valve cusps or leaflets (rcc, lcc) appear faint in young patients. *Bottom panel.* Note the thin diastolic closure line and the normal box-like opening and closing profile of the normal aortic cusps (insert sketch). Measure aortic root (Ao) diameter at end-diastole (blue line #1). Note also that the left atrial (LA) dimensions are largest during systole. Measure and record the largest LA dimensions at end-systole (yellow line #2). *IVS: interventricular septum; LV: left ventricle; ncc: non-coronary aortic cusp; PW: posterior wall; RA: right atrium; rcc: right coronary aortic cusp; RV: right ventricle.*

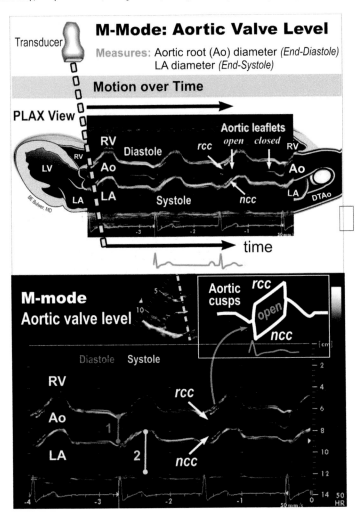

PLAX VIEW: M-MODE EXAMINATION OF THE MITRAL VALVE
Figure 6.13

Normal M-mode examination of the parasternal long-axis (PLAX) view at the level of the mitral valve leaflets. **Top panel.** Panoramic perspective of the M-mode display. **Middle panel.** Note the cyclical pattern of mitral leaflet behavior. This reflects transmitral LV inflow filling patterns, with abrupt opening in early diastole (E), partial closure during diastasis, and secondary opening during late diastole (A) because of left atrial contraction. See Figures 7.14–7.16. The EF slope reflects the speed of anterior mitral leaflet (AML) closure. This pattern is significantly altered in mitral stenosis (Figure 6.26), becoming boxlike. Posterior mitral leaflet (PML) movement essentially mirrors that of the anterior leaflet. *aml: anterior mitral valve leaflet; pml: posterior mitral valve leaflet; ivs: interventricular septum; pw: posterior wall (more correctly—the inferolateral wall) of the left ventricle.*

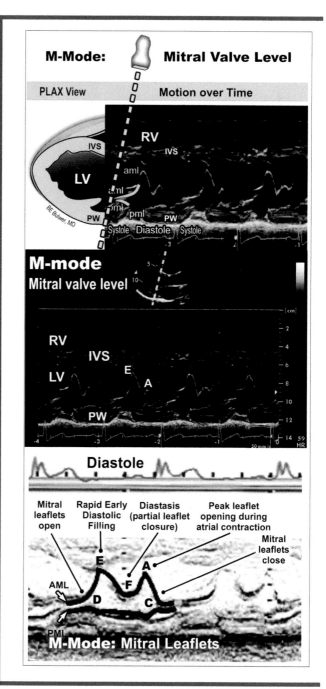

PLAX VIEW: M-MODE EXAMINATION AT THE LV LEVEL AND MEASUREMENTS

Figure 6.14

Normal M-mode examination of the parasternal long-axis (PLAX) view at the level of the mid-left ventricle (just distal to the tips of the mitral valve leaflets). Orient the M-mode cursor perpendicular to the long axis of the left ventricle (LV) at the level of the mitral valve chordae—just distal to the tips of the mitral leaflets.

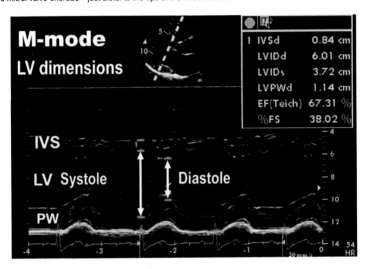

M-mode images exhibit superior temporal resolution compared to 2D images, but variations in cardiac topography and morphology frequently lead to off-axis measurements, thereby resulting in measurement errors. Therefore, for optimal LV systolic function assessment (Figure 6.18), it is important to align and record LV dimensions with the M-mode cursor perpendicular to the long axis of the LV at the level of the minor (or short) axis, corresponding to the level of the mitral leaflet tips.

Measure LV ventricular wall thicknesses—septum (IVS) and "posterior" (PW) walls—during diastole (Figure 6.14). Measure the LV internal diameters during systole (LVIDs) and diastole (LVIDd). Measures of LV systolic function, e.g., the ejection fraction and fractional shortening, can be estimated from M-mode measurements, assuming a geometrically normal LV (Figures 6.18–6.20). Echocardiography instruments can automatically estimate the LV ejection fraction (LVEF) using the Teichholz formula, but this method is very unreliable and therefore not recommended.

The LVEF is the percentage of blood ejected from the LV during each cardiac cycle. It is routinely estimated subjectively ("Eyeball" LVEF), or quantitatively (Figures 6.19, 6.20), and is defined as: $[(EDV - ESV) / EDV] \times 100\%$, where EDV is the end-diastolic volume and ESV is the end-systolic volume.

PLAX VIEW: 2D AND LINEAR MEASUREMENTS
Figure 6.15

Linear dimensions measured using the parasternal long-axis (PLAX) view. These are preferred to the M-mode measures (in Figures 6.12–6.14) because 2D images minimize off-axis measurements even with distorted ventricular geometry. *Top left.* Optimize and record a video loop of the parasternal long-axis (PLAX) view. Scroll through frames and select an end-systolic frame (with the smallest LV diameter), and measure the left atrial (LA) diameter as shown. *Top right.* Measure the aortic (Ao) root diameter at the level of the aortic valve annulus (see Figure 6.27). *Bottom left.* Scroll and select end-diastolic frame (with the largest LV diameter), and measure LV ventricular wall thicknesses—septum (IVS) and "posterior" (PW) walls, and the LV internal diameter during diastole (LVIDd). *Bottom right.* Scroll and select end-systolic frame, and measure the LV internal diameter during systole (LVIDs).

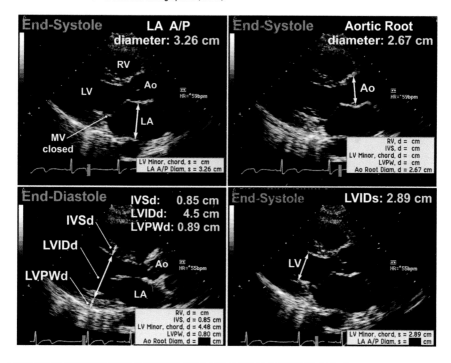

The parasternal long-axis (PLAX) window is the recommended site for obtaining linear measures of LV wall dimensions (Figures 6.12–6.15). M-mode measurement, because of its superior temporal resolution, can complement 2D measurements especially when there is need to distinguish the endocardium from ventricular wall trabeculae, chordae tendinae, or false tendons. Linear M-mode or 2D measurements can be recorded using both PLAX and PSAX views of the LV at the chordae level, and such measures are used to quantify various parameters of global ventricular function (Figures 6.18–6.20) and (Tables 12.1–12.3).

LV dimensions measured by 2D are generally smaller than the corresponding M-mode measurements in the same patient, with the upper limit of normal LVIDd of 5.2 versus 5.5 cm, and for fractional shortening (FS % = [LVIDd − LVIDs] / LVIDd), the lower limits of normal FS of 0.18 versus 0.25. A normal LV ejection fraction (LVEF) is considered ≥55%.

The normal range of LV size, volumes, and function for both males and females, indexed to height and body surface area (BSA), are listed in Figures 6.18, 6.20, 6.21 and Tables 12.1 to 12.3 .

PLAX VIEW: COLOR FLOW DOPPLER EXAMINATION OF THE MITRAL AND AORTIC VALVES
Figure 6.16

Normal color flow Doppler examination of the aortic and mitral valve on the PLAX view. Despite the nonparallel alignment of flow direction to the transducer, the blue-away, red-toward ("BART") pattern of flow is readily discerned.

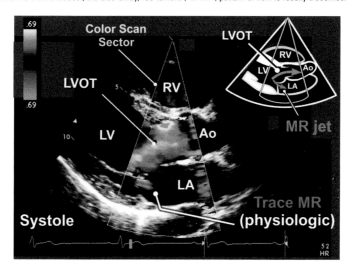

Figure 6.17

Color flow Doppler examination of the mitral valve on PLAX *(top panels)* and apical four-chamber (A4C) views *(lower panels)* comparing color flow jets of mitral regurgitation (MR). Color gain setting is important and has a major impact on the appearance and therefore the visual estimation of the valvular regurgitant jets (see Figure 6.25).

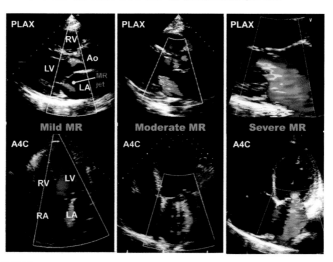

AN APPROACH TO ASSESSMENT OF CARDIAC STRUCTURE AND FUNCTION—BEGINNING WITH THE PLAX VIEW

The primary purpose of the echocardiographic examination is to assess and record cardiac structure and function. As echocardiography is primarily a visual specialty, it follows that visual assessment (qualitative), and measures based thereon (semiquantitative), remain the cornerstone of its interpretation and analysis. Such "eyeball" assessment or visual estimates of cardiac structure and function are routinely used and reported in clinical practice. They are reliable and reproducible in experienced hands   Figures 6.19, 6.22 .

However, as echocardiographic parameters play important roles in cardiovascular diagnosis, risk stratification, management, and prognosis, quantification of such findings is necessary. Therefore, in addition to subjective or qualitative assessment, semiquantitative and quantitative measures of cardiac function should be an integral part of echocardiographic interpretation, analysis, and reporting   Figures 6.18–6.34, 12.3 .

- Assess cardiac structure and function as the examination proceeds.
- Use all available windows and views to gather a comprehensive assessment of cardiac structure and function.
- Be systematic. Use a logical sequence, e.g., following the normal blood flow pattern, is good practice.
- Assessment of ventricular function—especially the left ventricular (LV) systolic function   Figures 6.18–6.23 —is perhaps the most common request in echocardiography. This should be assessed using orthogonal views. Initially, this is a qualitative assessment, but measurement using methods recommended by expert bodies should be performed.
- Whenever pathology is detected during the examination, perform the necessary measures and assessments, including additional views and performing the recommended measurements   Figures 6.18–6.34, 6.43, 6.44, 6.48 .
- As coronary artery disease is the most common cause of ventricular wall motion abnormalities, correlate such wall motion abnormalities with the corresponding coronary artery territory   Figure 6.23 .
- When evidence of valvular heart disease, e.g., valvular regurgitation or stenosis, is present, this requires a comprehensive assessment, not only of the valvular lesion, but also its impact on overall cardiac function   Figures 6.24–6.29, 6.34, 6.43, 6.44, 6.48 .
- A comprehensive assessment of valvular lesions should be performed by an expert sonographer/cardiologist.

PLAX VIEW SURVEY: NORMAL AND ABNORMAL FINDINGS

Table 6.1 PARASTERNAL LONG-AXIS (PLAX) VIEW: THE EXAMINATION SURVEY

Sequential survey (by flow sequence)	Parasternal long-axis (PLAX) view	
	Structural: on 2D, 3D, or M-mode	Functional and hemodynamic Doppler
	Assess	
Left atrium (LA)	LA CAVITY SIZE • Size: Normal, increased, decreased • LA enlargement: mild, moderate, severe (note post cardiac transplant, cor triatriatum) LA CAVITY APPEARANCE • Mass: most commonly myxoma, thrombus (clot) • "Smoke" (spontaneous echocontrast) MEASURE AND RECORD By 2D and M-mode • LA size (systole) [Figs. 6.12, 6.15] LA DIMENSIONS, AREAS, VOLUMES [Figs. 6.12, 6.15, 6.30] ; [Table 12.6]	LA PHASIC DYNAMICS • LA acts as "reservoir-conduit-pump" [Figs. 7.14, 7.15] • Loss of atrial "pump" (atrial fibrillation) • Diastolic collapse of LA free wall (pericardial tamponade) [Fig. 6.33]
Mitral valve (MV)	MV STRUCTURE [Figs. 6.24, 6.61] **Mitral leaflets:** mobility, thickness, and closure (coaptation): • **Mitral valve apparatus** includes: mitral annulus, chordae tendinae, anterolateral papillary muscle, and LV wall • **Leaflet vegetation:** location, size, mobility ± perforation (suspect infective endocarditis) • **MAC (mitral annular calcification)** especially of posterior annulus MV LEAFLET MOBILITY • **Excessive movement of one or both leaflets:** Mitral valve prolapse (MVP) [Fig. 6.24], leaflet flail with chordal or papillary muscle rupture	MV DYNAMICS • **Systolic anterior motion (SAM)** of the mitral valve ± dynamic LVOT obstruction (confirm on M-mode) • **Diastolic fluttering of anterior mitral leaflet (AML)** ± premature MV closure in aortic regurgitation (AR) MITRAL REGURGITATION (MR) • Assess etiology • Estimate severity: mild, moderate, severe [Fig. 6.25] MITRAL STENOSIS (MS) • Assess etiology • Estimate severity: mild, moderate, severe [Fig. 6.26] MITRAL VALVE SCORING CRITERIA IN MS (Wilkins score): for balloon valvuloplasty decision making and outcomes

(continues)

Table 6.1 PARASTERNAL LONG-AXIS (PLAX) VIEW: THE EXAMINATION SURVEY *(continued)*

Sequential survey (by flow sequence)	Parasternal long-axis (PLAX) view	
	Structural: on 2D, 3D, or M-mode	Functional and hemodynamic Doppler
	MV PROLAPSE criteria Fig. 6.24 : • Superior displacement of both leaflets ≥2 mm above plane of mitral annuls • Leaflet thickening (>5 mm) in diastole • ± Mitral regurgitation (MR) • ± Chordal rupture/leaflet flail • PLAX and A3C views preferred to A4C view • **Restricted leaflet motion** ("doming"), thickened leaflets, "hockey-stick" anterior leaflet with mitral stenosis (MS) Fig. 6.26 • Prosthetic MV: mechanical vs. bioprosthetic; normal vs. abnormal function; valvular and paravalvular dysfunction	• Leaflet mobility (1–4) • Subvalvular thickening (chordae + papillary muscles [1–4]) • Valve leaflet thickening: margins→entire leaflet (1–4) • Calcification: mild→extensive (1–4) • Total score of <8 = better outcomes with percutaneous balloon dilatation of the mitral valve
Left ventricle (LV)	LV CAVITY SIZE • Normal or dilated: mild, moderate, severe Fig. 6.20 , Table 12.1 • Decreased LV cavity size (volume depletion; also check IVC collapsibility index on subcostal view) Table 8.1 • Decreased LV cavity (because of cavity obliteration (markedly thickened walls) LV WALL THICKNESS: Figs. 6.14, 6.15 • **LV hypertrophy** (≥12 mm in adults) including hypertrophic cardiomyopathy (most commonly asymmetric septal hypertrophy; discrete upper septal hypertrophy (DUSH) or thickening (DUST)	LV SYSTOLIC FUNCTION ASSESSMENT • Summary measures Figs. 6.18–6.23 LV EJECTION FRACTION • Figs. 6.18–6.20 , Table 12.2 • "Eyeball estimate" of LV ejection fraction (LVEF) used in routine practice Figs. 6.19, 6.20 • Biplane method of disks (Simpson's rule) Fig. 6.20 LV WALL MOTION and WALL THICKENING • Wall motion score (WMS) and WMS Index Figs. 6.21, 6.22 . • Correlate with corresponding coronary artery blood supply Figs. 6.10, 6.23

Table 6.1 PARASTERNAL LONG-AXIS (PLAX) VIEW: THE EXAMINATION SURVEY *(continued)*

Sequential survey (by flow sequence)	Parasternal long-axis (PLAX) view	
	Structural: on 2D, 3D, or M-mode	Functional and hemodynamic Doppler
	LV WALL STRUCTURE • LV walls visualized and assessed: anteroseptal and inferolateral ("posterior") walls Figs. 6.10, 6.21, 6.22 • "Speckled" myocardium in infiltrative disease, e.g., amyloidosis • LV aneurysm or pseudoaneurysm— especially of posterior wall LV MASSES • LV masses, e.g., thrombus, tumor • LV opacification using contrast agents often necessary MEASURE AND RECORD By 2D and M-mode • LVIDd, LVIDs, IVSd, PWTd Figs. 6.14, 6.15 • Calculate fractional shortening (FS); LVEF by Teichholz (unreliable) LV DIMENSIONS, AREAS, VOLUMES: Figs. 6.14, 6.15, 6.18–6.22 ; Tables 12.1–12.3	ASSESS LV DIASTOLIC FUNCTION (primarily using apical 4-chamber Doppler measures Figs. 7.14–7.25 ; Table 7.1 ; enlarged left atrium: a feature of diastolic dysfunction
Interventricular septum (IVS)	INTERVENTRICULAR SEPTUM Fig. 6.34 • Membranous • Perimembranous • Muscular/trabecular (inlet septum) • Muscular/trabecular (outlet septum) VENTRICULAR SEPTAL DEFECT (VSD) Fig. 6.34 • Anatomical categorization— membranous, perimembranous, or muscular (trabecular) • Size: small, moderate, large • Restrictive vs. nonrestrictive IVS FLATTENING (D-shaped septum on PSAX views) Figs. 6.31, 6.32 • Flattening in systole: RV pressure overload states • Flattening in systole and diastole: RV pressure and volume overload	ABNORMAL/PARADOXICAL SEPTAL MOTION Figs. 6.31–6.34 • Left bundle branch block (LBBB) • Pacemaker • Post heart surgery • RV pressure and volume overload states—pulmonary hypertension, L-to-R shunts, e.g., secundum ASD • Constrictive pericarditis—"septal bounce" DYSSYNCHRONY • LV dyssynchrony (confirm on M-mode) VSD Fig. 6.34 • Assess on color flow, PW, and CW Doppler and using other views • Categorize physiology: restrictive vs. nonrestrictive VSD • Assess pulmonary-to-systemic flow ratio (Qp:Qs)

(continues)

Table 6.1 PARASTERNAL LONG-AXIS (PLAX) VIEW: THE EXAMINATION SURVEY *(continued)*

Sequential survey (by flow sequence)	Parasternal long-axis (PLAX) view	
	Structural: on 2D, 3D, or M-mode	Functional and hemodynamic Doppler
LV outflow tract (LVOT)	LVOT OBSTRUCTION • Septal hypertrophy in hypertrophic cardiomyopathy (HCM) • Severe LV hypertrophy (LVH) • Systolic anterior motion (SAM) of the anterior mitral valve leaflet in HCM • Discrete upper septal hypertrophy (DUSH) • Subvalvular membrane • Prolapsed aortic dissection flap • Aortic cusp, valve prolapse • Dehiscence of aortic valve prosthesis with prolapse	DOPPLER ASSESSMENT • Color flow, PW, and CW Doppler: for signs of accelerated flow with SAM or subvalvular membrane • Measure LVOT diameter 1 cm proximal to AV leaflets (for calculation of stroke volume/cardiac output or for aortic valve area calculation in aortic stenosis [AS]) Figs. 4.15, 6.27–6.29
Aortic valve (AV)	AV STRUCTUR Figs. 6.9, 6.12, 6.27–6.29 • Observe the normal trileaflet (cusps) structure identify: leaflets, annulus, sinus of Valsalva, aortic root • **Thickened and echoreflective "calcified" AV leaflets ± annulus** in aortic sclerosis (elderly), aortic stenosis (AS) Fig. 6.29 • **Valvular thickening and systolic doming** with bicuspid aortic valve (BAV); quadricuspid and unicuspid variants • Aortic dimensions Fig. 6.27 • **Mobile** vegetation(s) ± leaflet perforation in infective endocarditis, papillary fibroelastoma, Lambl's excrescences • Prosthetic AV valve: mechanical vs. bioprosthetic • **Supravalvular thickening** MEASURE AND RECORD By 2D and M-mode Figs. 6.9, 6.12, 6.27 • **Aortic diameters** at various levels: annulus, sinus of Valsalva, sinotubular junction, ascending aorta, descending thoracic aorta (DTAo)	PHASIC BEHAVIOR (ROOT) • Note normal systolic anterior motion of the aortic root and proximal ascending aorta (movement toward sternum) Fig. 6.12 AORTIC REGURGITATION (AR) • Assess etiology • Estimate severity: mild, moderate, severe Fig. 6.28 AORTIC STENOSIS (AS) • Assess etiology • Estimate severity: mild, moderate, severe Figs. 4.15, 6.29, 10.2

Table 6.1 PARASTERNAL LONG-AXIS (PLAX) VIEW: THE EXAMINATION SURVEY *(continued)*

Sequential survey (by flow sequence)	Parasternal long-axis (PLAX) view	
	Structural: on 2D, 3D, or M-mode	Functional and hemodynamic Doppler
Aortic root; Proximal ascending aorta (Ao)	• Aortic root dilatation: in hypertension, Marfan syndrome, bicuspid aortic valve disease (BAV) • Atherosclerotic plaque in the ascending aorta • Sinus of Valsalva aneurysm • Intimal flap (aortic dissection) in aortic root or ascending aorta ± aortic leaflet prolapse (new onset AR) • MEASURE AND RECORD: by 2D and M-mode Fig. 6.27 **Aortic diameters** at sinus of Valsalva, sinotubular junction, ascending aorta, descending thoracic aorta (DTAo)	AORTIC ANEURYSMS: Aortic root, ascending, arch, descending thoracic, abdominal • ± Aortic regurgitation (AR) with Doppler findings SUPRAVALVULAR AORTIC STENOSIS (AS) • Assess etiology • Estimate severity: mild, moderate, severe AORTIC DISSECTION (AD) • Color flow Doppler and spectral Doppler: new onset AR (with aortic root dissection) • ± Pericardial tamponade physiology (Doppler)
Right ventricle (RV)	RV/RVOT CAVITY SIZE Figs. 6.31, 6.32 ; Table 12.5 • Size: normal, increased, or decreased • Eyeball estimate: RV/RVOT cavity size • RV dilatation in RV pressure and volume overload states, e.g., right heart failure; primary and secondary pulmonary hypertension; secundum ASD RV/RVOT FREE WALL • Thickened in chronic overload states, e.g., chronic pulmonary hypertension RV MASSES • Thrombus (clot) • Tumor • Pacemaker or defibrillator wire MEASURE AND RECORD By 2D and M-mode • RV diameter Figs. 6.14, 6.15 RV DIMENSIONS, AREAS, VOLUMES: Figs. 6.31, 6.32 ; Tables 12.4, 12.5	RV SYSTOLIC FUNCTION • "Eyeball" estimate of RV systolic function RV FUNCTION MEASURES Figs. 6.31, 6.32 ; Table 12.4 • RV diameters • RV diastolic area • RV systolic area • RV fractional area change • Systolic dysfunction (confirm in A4C and subcostal views impaired contractility, e.g., in RV pressure and volume overload states • Paradoxical septal motion: IVS flattening "D-shaped" during systole (RV pressure overload); during systole and diastole (RV pressure and volume overload) RV/RVOT FREE WALL • Diastolic collapse with pericardial tamponade—confirm on M-mode and Doppler Fig. 6.33

(continues)

Table 6.1 PARASTERNAL LONG-AXIS (PLAX) VIEW:
THE EXAMINATION SURVEY *(continued)*

Sequential survey (by flow sequence)	Parasternal long-axis (PLAX) view	
	Structural: on 2D, 3D, or M-mode	Functional and hemodynamic Doppler
Pericardium (fibrous)	STRUCTURE: circumferential with oblique and transverse sinuses Fig. 6.33 • Appearance: normal, abnormal: thickening, calcification, effusion EFFUSION • Pericardial effusion—distinguish from L pleural effusion by comparing relationship to descending thoracic aorta • Site: localized, circumferential • Echolucency: homogenous, heterogenous ± opacities, stranding, masses • Abnormal IVS movements (septal bounce) • Pericardial swinging EFFUSION SIZE (linear measurement by 2D or M-mode) For circumferential effusion • Trace-to-mild (<50 ml → < 0.5 cm thick) • Mild-to-moderate (50–250 ml → >0.5 to <2 cm thick) moderate • Large (>500 ml → >2 cm thick)	TAMPONADE PHYSIOLOGY (tamponade: a clinical diagnosis) **2D and M-mode findings with increasing severity** • RA ± LA systolic collapse • RVOT diastolic collapse • LVOT diastolic collapse TAMPONADE PHYSIOLOGY **Doppler findings** • Exaggerated respirophasic MV and TV inflow patterns • A4C: PW Doppler-MV: >15% variation • A4C: PW Doppler-TV: >25% variation CONSTRICTIVE PHYSIOLOGY **2D and M-mode** • Thickened pericardium with adhesions ± tethering • Dyskinetic septal and wall movements • Usually normal LV function (compared to restrictive cardiomyopathy that it resembles clinically)
Descending thoracic aorta (DTAo)	VIEWS Fig. 6.27 • Dissection flap in descending thoracic aorta • Intra-aortic balloon pump • Dilatation (do not confuse with dilated coronary sinus)	• PW Doppler—rarely applied because of large Doppler angle • Descending thoracic aorta best examined by transesophageal echocardiography (TEE)
Coronary sinus	• Dilated chamber—if marked, should raise possibility of persistent L superior vena cava (PLSVC) • Cardiac hardware, e.g., defibrillator wire • MV support device to treat MR	• Confirm PLSVC by agitated saline "bubble" study injected into L arm vein. This opacifies coronary sinus before it enters RA.

OVERVIEW: VENTRICULAR SYSTOLIC FUNCTION ASSESSMENT

Figure 6.18

Summary measures of left ventricular systolic function.

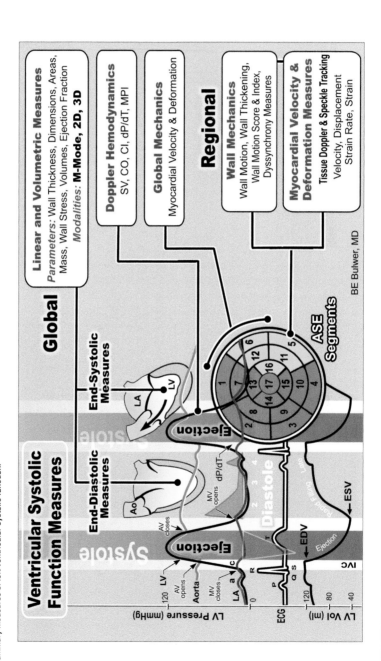

QUALITATIVE AND SEMIQUANTITATIVE MEASURES OF LV SYSTOLIC FUNCTION: MOVEMENT OF MYOCARDIAL WALLS

Grading Regional Wall Motion

Left ventricular myocardial segment scores are assigned based on two qualitative measures of ventricular wall behavior during systole: (i) wall movement (contraction), and (ii) wall thickening Figures 6.21, 6.22 . Graded scores of contractility of the individual segments range from a normal score of 1 to a worst score of 5.

A dysfunctional segment of the myocardium thickens less (or becomes thinner) during systole. A segment that exhibits noticeable reduction in contractility is *hypokinetic* and assigned a score of 2. A segment that barely moves or thickens during systole is *akinetic* (score = 3). *Dyskinetic* myocardium moves paradoxically during systole (score = 4). *Aneurysmal* myocardial segments tend to balloon out during systole (score = 5). The integrated wall motion score is the sum of the scores divided by the number of scored segments. A wall score index of 1 indicates normality. Larger scores reflect more severe degrees of systolic dysfunction Figures 6.21, 6.22 .

Normal ventricular walls thicken during systole—a manifestation of myocardial fiber shortening—as both ventricles contract. Ventricular systolic contraction is accompanied by a reduction in ventricular cavity size that can be visually assessed as visually as normal, reduced, or hyperdynamic.

Normally, 60–70% of ventricular end-diastolic volume is ejected during each cardiac cycle Figures 6.19, 6.20 ; Table 12.2 .

Reduction of LV systolic function, as assessed by the LV ejection fraction (LVEF), can be estimated to the nearest 5 or 10% by an experienced observer Figure 6.19 .

≥ 55%	• Normal
40 − 55%	• Mildly reduced
30 − 40%	• Moderately reduced
< 30%	• Severely reduced
> 70%	• Hyperdynamic

A LVEF exceeding 75% appears as near obliteration of the LV cavity when viewed on the parasternal and apical windows. As visual estimates of LVEF ("eyeball EF") by experienced personnel correlate well with quantitative measures of EF, this is therefore a practical first step during the routine echocardiographic examination.

VISUAL ESTIMATE OF LV EJECTION FRACTION: "EYEBALL EF"
Figure 6.19

Views illustrating subjective visual "eyeball" estimates of left ventricular ejection fraction (LVEF) as the examination proceeds. *A2C: apical two-chamber view; A3C: apical three-chamber view; A4C: apical four-chamber view; ALAX: apical long-axis view; PSAX-PML: parasternal short-axis view—papillary muscle level.*

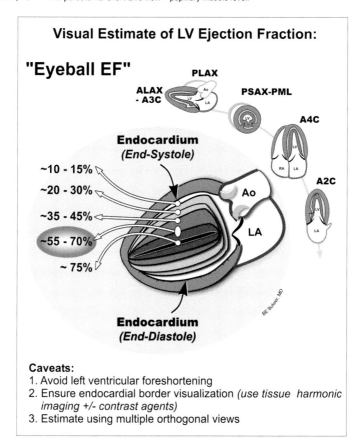

Eyeball LVEF is routinely estimated as the examination proceeds. This is reliable and reproducible, and improves with training and experience. Note that it is the endocardial border, not the external epicardial border, that should be visually tracked to estimate the LVEF. As the LV endocardial border moves or "contracts" to a much greater extent than the outer myocardium, failure to clearly visualize the endocardial border can lead to significant underestimation of LVEF. Left ventricular opacification using contrast agents should be used to facilitate endocardial border delineation Figures 6.20, 6.21 ; Table 12.2 .

GLOBAL MEASURES OF LEFT VENTRICULAR SYSTOLIC FUNCTION

Figure 6.20

Global measures of left ventricular (LV) systolic function (see Table 12.2).

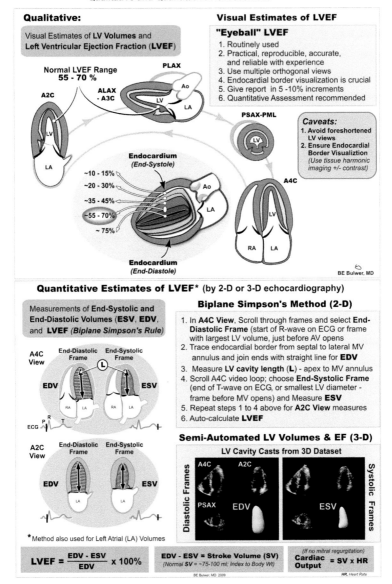

Global LV Systolic Function: Volumetric Measures
Qualitative and Quantitative Asssessment

Qualitative:

Visual Estimates of **LV Volumes** and
Left Ventricular Ejection Fraction (LVEF)

Normal LVEF Range
55 - 70 %

PLAX
A2C
ALAX
- A3C
Ao
LV
LA

LV
LA

Endocardium
(End-Systole)

~10 - 15%
~20 - 30%
~35 - 45%
~55 - 70%
~ 75%

Endocardium
(End-Diastole)

PSAX-PML
LV

Ao
LA

A4C
LV
RA LA

Visual Estimates of LVEF

"Eyeball" LVEF
1. Routinely used
2. Practical, reproducible, accurate, and reliable with experience
3. Use multiple orthogonal views
4. Endocardial border visualization is crucial
5. Give report in 5 -10% increments
6. Quantitative Assessment recommended

Caveats:
1. Avoid foreshortened LV views
2. Ensure Endocardial Border Visualiztion
(Use tissue harmonic imaging +/- contrast)

BE Bulwer, MD

Quantitative Estimates of LVEF* (by 2-D or 3-D echocardiography)

Measurements of **End-Systolic** and
End-Diastolic Volumes (ESV, EDV,
and **LVEF** *(Biplane Simpson's Rule)*

A4C View — End-Diastolic Frame / End-Systolic Frame — L
EDV / ESV
RA LA / RA LA
ECG — P R T

A2C View — End-Diastolic Frame / End-Systolic Frame
EDV / ESV
LA / LA

*Method also used for Left Atrial (LA) Volumes

Biplane Simpson's Method (2-D)

1. In **A4C View**, Scroll through frames and select **End-Diastolic Frame** (start of R-wave on ECG or frame with largest LV volume, just before AV opens)
2. Trace endocardial border from septal to lateral MV annulus and join ends with straight line for **EDV**
3. Measure **LV cavity length (L)** - apex to MV annulus
4. Scroll A4C video loop; choose **End-Systolic Frame** (end of T-wave on ECG, or smallest LV diameter - frame before MV opens) and Measure **ESV**
5. Repeat steps 1 to 4 above for **A2C View** measures
6. Auto-calculate **LVEF**

Semi-Automated LV Volumes & EF (3-D)

LV Cavity Casts from 3D Dataset

Diastolic Frames
A4C A2C
PSAX EDV

Systolic Frames
ESV

$$LVEF = \frac{EDV - ESV}{EDV} \times 100\%$$

EDV - ESV = Stroke Volume (SV)
(Normal SV = ~75-100 ml; Index to Body Wt)

(If no mitral regurgitation)
Cardiac Output = SV x HR

HR, Heart Rate

BE Bulwer, MD 2009

REGIONAL MEASURES OF LEFT VENTRICULAR SYSTOLIC FUNCTION
Figure 6.21

Regional measures of left ventricular (LV) systolic function.

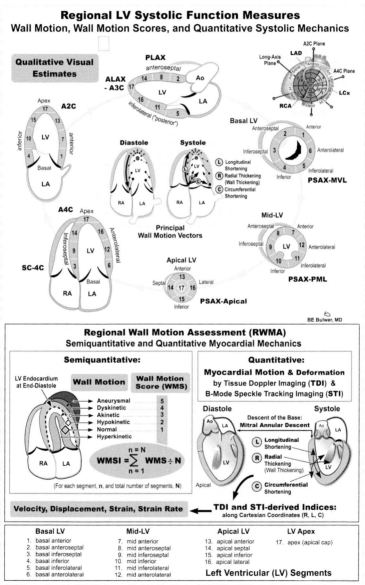

PLAX, Parasternal Long-Axis; **PSAX-MVL**, Parasternal Short-Axis (Mitral Valve Level); **PSAX-PML**, PSAX (Papillary Muscle or Mid-LV Level). **PSAX-Apical**, PSAX (Apical level); **A4C**, Apical 4-Chamber View; **A2C**, Apical 2-Chamber View; **A3C / ALAX**, Apical 3-Chamber or Apical Long-Axis View

REGIONAL WALL MOTION ASSESSMENT
Figure 6.22

Left ventricular function: regional wall motion assessment (RWMA).

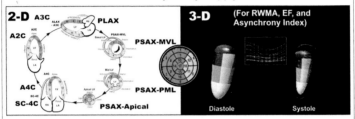

Regional Wall Motion Assessment (RWMA)
Semiquantitative / Quantitative (2-D and 3-D)

1. Acquire and Record Video Loops (Standard Exam Protocol)

2. Use 16- or 17-Segment ASE/AHA/ACC LV Segmentation Model and Correlate with Coronary Artery Supply

3. Observe Systolic LV Wall Motion in each view (Video loop) and Score each segment, with special focus on:

NORMAL

1. Endocardial Motion

2. Wall Thickening

(30 to 70% ↑ systolic endocardial thickening)

4. Record Wall Motion Scores and WMS Index (automated)

5. Avoid foreshortened LV views and beware pseudodyskinesis

BE Bulwer, MD

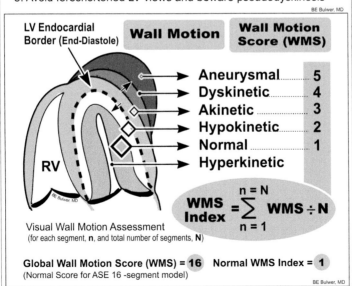

LV Endocardial Border (End-Diastole)	Wall Motion	Wall Motion Score (WMS)
	Aneurysmal	5
	Dyskinetic	4
	Akinetic	3
	Hypokinetic	2
	Normal	1
RV	Hyperkinetic	

$$\text{WMS Index} = \sum_{n=1}^{n=N} \text{WMS} \div N$$

Visual Wall Motion Assessment
(for each segment, **n**, and total number of segments, **N**)

Global Wall Motion Score (WMS) = **16**   Normal WMS Index = **1**
(Normal Score for ASE 16 -segment model)

BE Bulwer, MD

CORONARY ARTERY TERRITORIES AND VENTRICULAR SEGMENTS
Figure 6.23

Coronary artery territories, imaging planes, and corresponding left ventricular (LV) segments. Where pertinent, the standard echocardiographic views of the left ventricle and their corresponding coronary supply are presented during discussions of each view. Compare with Figures 2.9, 6.10, 6.65, 7.13, 7.36, 7.42.

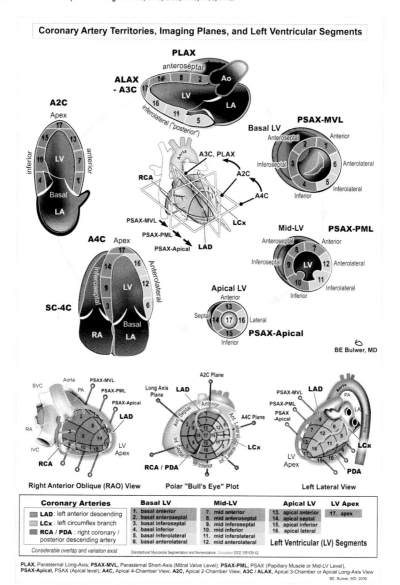

Coronary Artery Territories, Imaging Planes, and Left Ventricular Segments

BE Bulwer, MD

Coronary Arteries	Basal LV	Mid-LV	Apical LV	LV Apex
LAD : left anterior descending	1. basal anterior	7. mid anterior	13. apical anterior	17. apex
LCx : left circumflex branch	2. basal anteroseptal	8. mid anteroseptal	14. apical septal	
RCA / PDA : right coronary / posterior descending artery	3. basal inferoseptal	9. mid inferoseptal	15. apical inferior	
	4. basal inferior	10. mid inferior	16. apical lateral	
	5. basal inferolateral	11. mid inferolateral		
Considerable overlap and variation exist	6. basal anterolateral	12. mid anterolateral	**Left Ventricular (LV) Segments**	

Standardized Myocardial Segmentation and Nomenclature. Circulation 2002;105:539-42

PLAX, Parasternal Long-Axis; PSAX-MVL, Parasternal Short-Axis (Mitral Valve Level); PSAX-PML, PSAX (Papillary Muscle or Mid-LV Level); PSAX-Apical, PSAX (Apical level); A4C, Apical 4-Chamber View; A2C, Apical 2-Chamber View; A3C / ALAX, Apical 3-Chamber or Apical Long-Axis View

BE Bulwer, MD. 2009

THE MITRAL VALVE: ECHOCARDIOGRAPHIC VIEWS
Figure 6.24

Echocardiographic views of the mitral valve and mitral scallops.

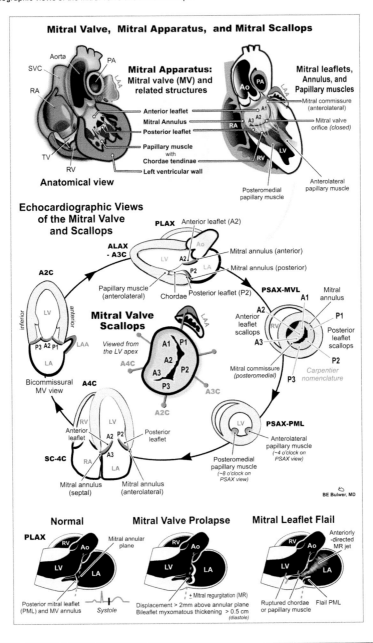

MITRAL REGURGITATION
Figure 6.25

Echocardiographic assessment of mitral regurgitation: a summary.

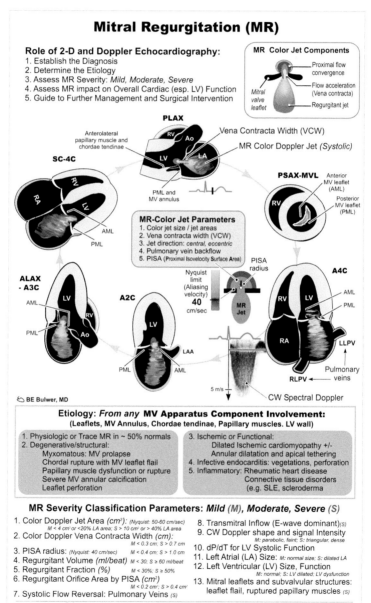

Mitral Regurgitation (MR)

Role of 2-D and Doppler Echocardiography:
1. Establish the Diagnosis
2. Determine the Etiology
3. Assess MR Severity: *Mild, Moderate, Severe*
4. Assess MR impact on Overall Cardiac (esp. LV) Function
5. Guide to Further Management and Surgical Intervention

MR Color Jet Components
- Proximal flow convergence
- Flow acceleration (Vena contracta)
- Regurgitant jet
- Mitral valve leaflet

PLAX — Vena Contracta Width (VCW)
MR Color Doppler Jet *(Systolic)*

Anterolateral papillary muscle and chordae tendinae

SC-4C

PML and MV annulus

PSAX-MVL — Anterior MV leaflet (AML) / Posterior MV leaflet (PML)

MR-Color Jet Parameters
1. Color jet size / jet areas
2. Vena contracta width (VCW)
3. Jet direction: *central, eccentric*
4. Pulmonary vein backflow
5. PISA (Proximal Isovelocity Surface Area)

PISA radius

Nyquist limit (Aliasing velocity) **40** cm/sec

MR Jet

A4C

ALAX - A3C

A2C

LLPV / RLPV — Pulmonary veins

CW Spectral Doppler

5 m/s

BE Bulwer, MD

Etiology: *From any* MV Apparatus Component Involvement:
(Leaflets, MV Annulus, Chordae tendinae, Papillary muscles. LV wall)

1. Physiologic or Trace MR in ~ 50% normals
2. Degenerative/structural:
   Myxomatous: MV prolapse
   Chordal rupture with MV leaflet flail
   Papillary muscle dysfunction or rupture
   Severe MV annular calcification
   Leaflet perforation
3. Ischemic or Functional:
   Dilated Ischemic cardiomyopathy +/-
   Annular dilatation and apical tethering
4. Infective endocarditis: vegetations, perforation
5. Inflammatory: Rheumatic heart disease
   Connective tissue disorders
   (e.g. SLE, scleroderma)

MR Severity Classification Parameters: *Mild (M), Moderate, Severe (S)*

1. Color Doppler Jet Area *(cm²)*: *(Nyquist: 50-60 cm/sec)* M < 4 cm² or <20% LA area; S > 10 cm² or > 40% LA area
2. Color Doppler Vena Contracta Width *(cm)*: M < 0.3 cm; S > 0.7 cm
3. PISA radius: *(Nyquist: 40 cm/sec)* M < 0.4 cm; S > 1.0 cm
4. Regurgitant Volume *(ml/beat)* M < 30; S ≥ 60 ml/beat
5. Regurgitant Fraction *(%)* M < 30%; S ≥ 50%
6. Regurgitant Orifice Area by PISA *(cm²)* M < 0.2 cm²; S > 0.4 cm²
7. Systolic Flow Reversal: Pulmonary Veins *(S)*
8. Transmitral Inflow (E-wave dominant)*(S)*
9. CW Doppler shape and signal Intensity M: parabolic, faint; S: triangular, dense
10. dP/dT for LV Systolic Function
11. Left Atrial (LA) Size: M: normal size; S: dilated LA
12. Left Ventricular (LV) Size, Function M: normal; S: LV dilated; LV dysfunction
13. Mitral leaflets and subvalvular structures: leaflet flail, ruptured papillary muscles *(S)*

Reference: ACC/AHA 2006 Guidelines for the Management of Patients with Valvular Heart Disease.
J Am Coll Cardiol. 2006 Aug 1;48(3):e1-148

MITRAL STENOSIS
Figure 6.26

Echocardiographic assessment of mitral stenosis: a summary.

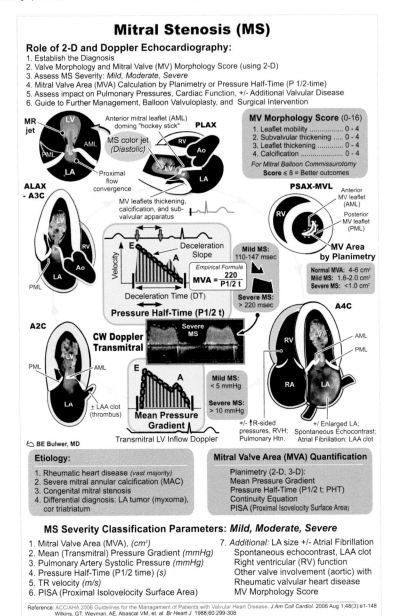

Mitral Stenosis (MS)

Role of 2-D and Doppler Echocardiography:
1. Establish the Diagnosis
2. Valve Morphology and Mitral Valve (MV) Morphology Score (using 2-D)
3. Assess MS Severity: *Mild, Moderate, Severe*
4. Mitral Valve Area (MVA) Calculation by Planimetry or Pressure Half-Time (P 1/2-time)
5. Assess impact on Pulmonary Pressures, Cardiac Function, +/- Additional Valvular Disease
6. Guide to Further Management, Balloon Valvuloplasty, and Surgical Intervention

MV Morphology Score (0-16)
1. Leaflet mobility .... 0 - 4
2. Subvalvular thickening ..... 0 - 4
3. Leaflet thickening .... 0 - 4
4. Calcification .... 0 - 4
For Mitral Balloon Commissurotomy
Score ≤ 8 = Better outcomes

MR jet · LV · Anterior mitral leaflet (AML) doming "hockey stick" · **PLAX** · MS color jet *(Diastolic)* · AML · RV · Ao · PML · LA · Proximal flow convergence

ALAX - A3C · MV leaflets thickening, calcification, and sub-valvular apparatus · LV · RV · Ao · LA · PML

PSAX-MVL · Anterior MV leaflet (AML) · Posterior MV leaflet (PML) · RV

MV Area by Planimetry
Normal MVA: 4-6 cm²
Mild MS: 1.6-2.0 cm²
Severe MS: <1.0 cm²

E · **Deceleration Slope** · A · Velocity · Deceleration Time (DT) · **Pressure Half-Time (P1/2 t)**

Empirical Formula
$$MVA = \frac{220}{P1/2\ t}$$

Mild MS: 110-147 msec
Severe MS: > 220 msec

A4C · RV · LV · AML · PML · RA · LA

A2C · LV · PML · AML · LA · ± LAA clot (thrombus)

CW Doppler Transmitral · Severe MS

E · A · **Mean Pressure Gradient** · Transmitral LV Inflow Doppler

Mild MS: < 5 mmHg
Severe MS: > 10 mmHg

+/- ↑R-sided pressures, RVH; Pulmonary Htn.
+/- Enlarged LA; Spontaneous Echocontrast; Atrial Fibrillation; LAA clot

⊘ BE Bulwer, MD

Etiology:
1. Rheumatic heart disease *(vast majority)*
2. Severe mitral annular calcification (MAC)
3. Congenital mitral stenosis
4. Differential diagnosis: LA tumor (myxoma), cor triatriatum

Mitral Valve Area (MVA) Quantification
Planimetry (2-D, 3-D):
Mean Pressure Gradient
Pressure Half-Time (P1/2 t; PHT)
Continuity Equation
PISA (Proximal Isovelocity Surface Area)

MS Severity Classification Parameters: *Mild, Moderate, Severe*

1. Mitral Valve Area (MVA), *(cm²)*
2. Mean (Transmitral) Pressure Gradient *(mmHg)*
3. Pulmonary Artery Systolic Pressure *(mmHg)*
4. Pressure Half-Time (P1/2 time) *(s)*
5. TR velocity *(m/s)*
6. PISA (Proximal Isolovelocity Surface Area)

7. *Additional:* LA size +/- Atrial Fibrillation
   Spontaneous echocontrast, LAA clot
   Right ventricular (RV) function
   Other valve involvement (aortic) with
   Rheumatic valvular heart disease
   MV Morphology Score

Reference: ACC/AHA 2006 Guidelines for the Management of Patients with Valvular Heart Disease. *J Am Coll Cardiol.* 2006 Aug 1;48(3):e1-148
Wilkins, GT, Weyman, AE, Abascal VM, et. al. *Br Heart J* 1988;60:299-308.

AORTA
Figure 6.27

Echocardiographic views of the aorta.

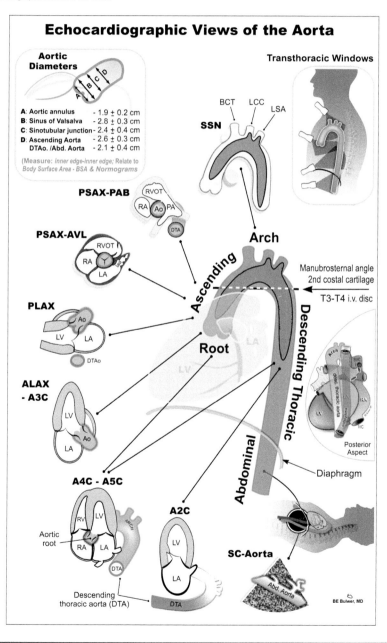

Echocardiographic Views of the Aorta

Aortic Diameters

A: Aortic annulus — 1.9 ± 0.2 cm
B: Sinus of Valsalva — 2.8 ± 0.3 cm
C: Sinotubular junction — 2.4 ± 0.4 cm
D: Ascending Aorta — 2.6 ± 0.3 cm
DTAo. /Abd. Aorta — 2.1 ± 0.4 cm

(Measure: Inner edge-inner edge; Relate to Body Surface Area - BSA & Normograms)

Transthoracic Windows

PSAX-PAB — RVOT, RA, Ao, PA, DTA

PSAX-AVL — RVOT, RA, LA

PLAX — Ao, LV, LA, DTAo

ALAX - A3C — LV, Ao, LA

A4C - A5C — RV, LV, RA, LA, ARCH, Aortic root, DTA

A2C — LV, LA, DTA

SC-Aorta — Abd. Aorta

SSN — BCT, LCC, LSA

Arch

Ascending

Root

Descending Thoracic

Abdominal

Manubrosternal angle
2nd costal cartilage
T3-T4 i.v. disc

Posterior Aspect

Diaphragm

Descending thoracic aorta (DTA)

BE Bulwer, MD

AORTIC REGURGITATION
Figure 6.28

Echocardiographic assessment of aortic regurgitation: a summary.

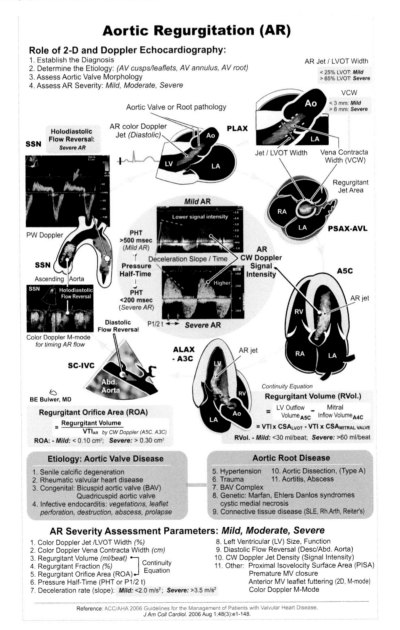

AORTIC STENOSIS
Figure 6.29

Echocardiographic assessment of aortic stenosis: a summary (see Figures 4.15, 10.2).

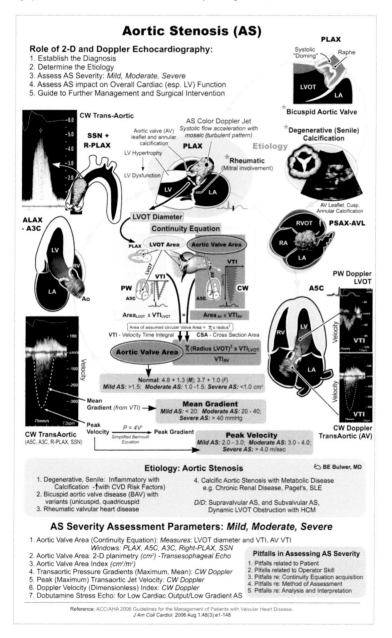

LEFT ATRIUM
Figure 6.30

Echocardiographic assessment of the left atrium (see Table 12.6).

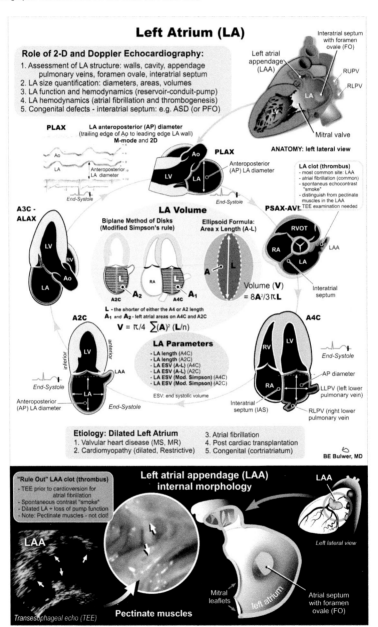

Left Atrium (LA)

Role of 2-D and Doppler Echocardiography:

1. Assessment of LA structure: walls, cavity, appendage pulmonary veins, foramen ovale, interatrial septum
2. LA size quantification: diameters, areas, volumes
3. LA function and hemodynamics (reservoir-conduit-pump)
4. LA hemodynamics (atrial fibrillation and thrombogenesis)
5. Congenital defects - interatrial septum: e.g. ASD (or PFO)

Interatrial septum with foramen ovale (FO)
Left atrial appendage (LAA)
RUPV
RLPV
LA
LV
Mitral valve
ANATOMY: left lateral view

PLAX LA anteroposterior (AP) diameter
(trailing edge of Ao to leading edge LA wall)
M-mode and 2D

Ao
LA
Anteroposterior LA diameter
End-Systole

PLAX
Ao
LV
LA
Anteroposterior (AP) LA diameter
End-Systole

LA clot (thrombus)
- most common site: LAA
- atrial fibrillation (common)
- spontaneus echocontrast "smoke"
- distinguish from pectinate muscles in the LAA
- TEE examination needed

A3C - ALAX
LV
RV
LA
Ao

LA Volume

Biplane Method of Disks (Modified Simpson's rule)
RA
A2
A2C
A1
A4C

Ellipsoid Formula: Area x Length (A-L)
A L

Volume (V) = $8A^2/3\pi L$

L - the shorter of either the A4 or A2 length
A_1 and A_2 - left atrial areas on A4C and A2C

$$V = \pi/4 \sum(A)^2 (L/n)$$

PSAX-AVL
RVOT
RA
LAA
LA
Interatrial septum

A2C
LV
LAA
LA
Anteroposterior (AP) LA diameter
End-Systole
inferior / anterior
End-Systole

LA Parameters
- LA length (A4C)
- LA length (A2C)
- LA ESV (A-L) (A4C)
- LA ESV (A-L) (A2C)
- LA ESV (Mod. Simpson) (A4C)
- LA ESV (Mod. Simpson) (A2C)

ESV: end systolic volume

A4C
RV
LV
End-Systole
AP diameter
RA
LLPV (left lower pulmonary vein)
Interatrial septum (IAS)
RLPV (right lower pulmonary vein)

Etiology: Dilated Left Atrium
1. Valvular heart disease (MS, MR)
2. Cardiomyopathy (dilated, Restrictive)
3. Atrial fibrillation
4. Post cardiac transplantation
5. Congenital (cortriatriatum)

BE Bulwer, MD

"Rule Out" LAA clot (thrombus)
- TEE prior to cardioversion for atrial fibrillation
- Spontaneous contrast "smoke"
- Dilated LA + loss of pump function
- Note: Pectinate muscles - not clot!

Left atrial appendage (LAA) internal morphology

LAA
LAA
Left lateral view
Mitral leaflets
left atrium
Atrial septum with foramen ovale (FO)

Transesophageal echo (TEE) **Pectinate muscles**

RIGHT VENTRICLE
Figure 6.31

Echocardiographic views of the right ventricle (see Tables 12.4, 12.5).

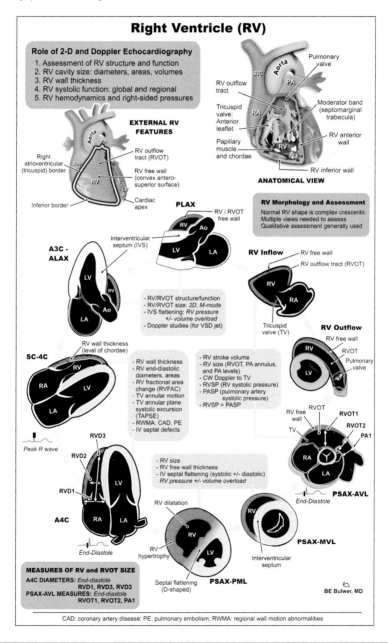

CAD: coronary artery disease; PE: pulmonary embolism; RWMA: regional wall motion abnormalities

RIGHT VENTRICLE
Figure 6.32

Echocardiographic assessment of the right ventricle (see Tables 12.4, 12.5).

RV Cavity Size, Wall Thickness, and Global RV Systolic Function
Qualitative and Quantitative Asssessment

Clinical Importance of RV Quantification	**RV quantification:** provides Important prognostic parameters in cardiopulmonary disease **RV size:** is sensitive to changes in afterload (pulmonary pressures and vascular resistance) **Increased RV afterload:** RV dilatation and RV hypertrophy **RV infarction and dysplasia / cardiomyopathy:** often manifests as RV dilatation and wall thinning

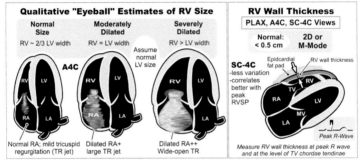

Qualitative "Eyeball" Estimates of RV Size

Normal Size — RV ~ 2/3 LV width
Moderately Dilated — RV = LV width
Severely Dilated — RV > LV width
Assume normal LV size

A4C

Normal RA; mild tricuspid regurgitation (TR jet)
Dilated RA+ large TR jet
Dilated RA++ Wide-open TR

RV Wall Thickness

PLAX, A4C, SC-4C Views

Normal: < 0.5 cm | 2D or M-Mode

SC-4C
-less variation
-correlates better with peak RVSP

Epicardial fat pad
RV wall thickness
Peak R-Wave

Measure RV wall thickness at peak R wave and at the level of TV chordae tendinae

Standard Linear Measures of RV Size

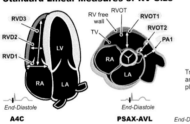

RVD3, RVD2, RVD1
RV free wall, RVOT, RVOT1, RVOT2, PA1, TV

End-Diastole — A4C
End-Diastole — PSAX-AVL

RV Fractional Area (RVA) Change

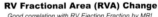

Good correlation with RV Ejection Fraction by MRI

RVA diastole
RVA systole

Tricuspid annular plane

A4C

End-Diastole — End-Systole

Other: **Tricuspid Annular Plane Systolic Excursion (TAPSE):** Normal (1.5 - 2.0 cm)
Regional Measures of RV Function: including wall motion abnormalities
Tissue Doppler Imaging (TDI): Tricuspid Annular Velocity
Myocardial Performance (Tei) Index   © BE Bulwer, MD

RV Global Systolic Function: Hemodynamics

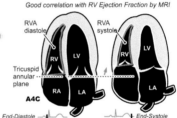

"Eyeball" Estimates

RV dilatation   RV hypertrophy
Flattening of the IV septum (D-shaped)
RV
LV

PSAX-PML

RV Volume Overload: Septal flattening (**diastole**)
RV Pressure Overload: Septal flattening (**systole**)
RV Pressure and Volume Overload:
    Septal flattening (**systole and diastole**)

RV Systolic Pressure

CW Doppler across TV

Tricuspid regurgitation (TR) jet   A4C

RVSP = PASP

Measure TR (Vmax)
Calculate RVSP, PASP

TR velocity profile

Bernoulli equation   Vmax

$RVSP = 4V_{TR-MAX}^2 + RA\ pressure$

RV Stroke Volume

Pulmonary Artery Diameter

CSA   RVOT
RA   Ao   PA

PSAX-PAB

$RV\ Stroke\ Volume = CSA_{PA} \times VTI_{PV}$

PV
Ao   PA

Pulmonary Valve VTI

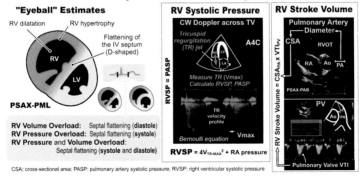

CSA; cross-sectional area; PASP: pulmonary artery systolic pressure; RVSP: right ventricular systolic pressure

PERICARDIUM
Figure 6.33

Echocardiographic assessment of the pericardium.

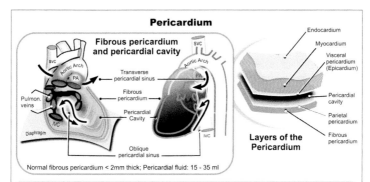

Pericardium

Fibrous pericardium and pericardial cavity

Layers of the Pericardium

Normal fibrous pericardium < 2mm thick; Pericardial fluid: 15 - 35 ml

Role of Echocardiography in Pericardial Disease
1. Diagnosis, etiology, severity assessment, and follow up in suspected pericardial disease
2. Tamponade physiology in patients with pericardial effusion
3. Constrictive physiology in patients with constriction, or effusive-constrictive process
4. Guide to pericardiocentesis

Echocardiographic Findings in Pericardial Disease: 2D, M-Mode, Doppler
1. Pericardial effusion: echolucency - localized or circumferential; +/- fibrin and fibrous strands, pericardial swinging; +/- **tamponade:** LA systolic collapse, RV diastolic collapse; +/- **constriction:** exaggerated LV and RV inflow patterns
2. Thickened pericardium +/- calcification, fibrous strands
3. Abnormal septal motion (septal "bounce")
4. Exaggerated mitral, tricuspid, pulmonary and IVC flows with respiration
5. Echocardiographic evidence of related or underlying disease

BE Bulwer, MD

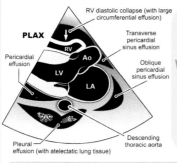

Pericardial Tamponade
Echo Features and Physiology

2D and M-mode findings
1. Pericardial effusion
2. RA inversion / collapse
3. Abnormal ventricular septal motion (ventricular interdependence)
4. RVOT diastolic collapse
5. LVOT diastolic collapse

Doppler findings
1. Exaggerated respiratory variation in flow velocity: MV and TV (A4C view)
2. Tamponade: variation > 40% *(normal variation* <15% at MV; < 25% at TV)
3. Right-sided reciprocal changes: TV, PV, IVC; IVC plethora - no collapse
4. Left-sided reciprocal changes: MV, AV, Pvv

AV: aortic valve; IVC: inferior vena cava; LVOT and RVOT: left and right ventricular outflow tract; PV: pulmon. valve; Pvv: pulmon. veins

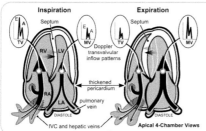

Pericardial Constrictive Physiology

2D and M-mode findings*
1. Thickened pericardium +/- calcification
2. Pericardial effusion +/- pericardial adhesions +/- echodensities in pericardial fluid
3. Abnormal septal motion (septal "bounce")
4. LV posterior wall diastolic flattening (M-mode

Doppler findings*
1. Differential ventricular filling patterns with respiration (PW Doppler to MV, TV, AV, PV, Pvv (non-compliant pericardium

* *Differentiate pericardial constriction from restrictive cardiomyopathy (similar symptoms/signs)*

INTERVENTRICULAR SEPTUM
Figure 6.34

Echocardiographic assessment of the interventricular septum.

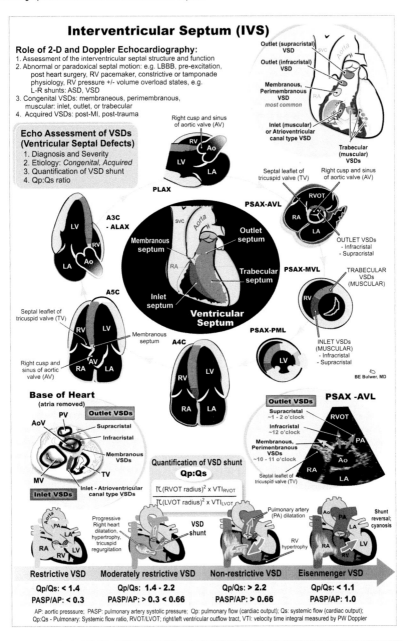

Interventricular Septum (IVS)

Role of 2-D and Doppler Echocardiography:
1. Assessment of the interventricular septal structure and function
2. Abnormal or paradoxical septal motion: e.g. LBBB, pre-excitation, post heart surgery, RV pacemaker, constrictive or tamponade physiology, RV pressure +/- volume overload states, e.g. L-R shunts: ASD, VSD
3. Congenital VSDs: membraneous, perimembranous, muscular: inlet, outlet, or trabecular
4. Acquired VSDs: post-MI, post-trauma

Echo Assessment of VSDs (Ventricular Septal Defects)
1. Diagnosis and Severity
2. Etiology: *Congenital, Acquired*
3. Quantification of VSD shunt
4. Qp:Qs ratio

Outlet (supracristal) VSD
Outlet (infracristal) VSD
Membranous, Perimembranous VSD *most common*
Inlet (muscular) or Atrioventricular canal type VSD
Trabecular (muscular) VSDs

Right cusp and sinus of aortic valve (AV)

PLAX

A3C - ALAX

A5C

Septal leaflet of tricuspid valve (TV)

Right cusp and sinus of aortic valve (AV)

Membranous septum

Outlet septum

Trabecular septum

Inlet septum

Ventricular Septum

Membranous septum

A4C

PSAX-AVL

OUTLET VSDs
- Infracristal
- Supracristal

Septal leaflet of tricuspid valve (TV)

Right cusp and sinus of aortic valve (AV)

PSAX-MVL

TRABECULAR VSDs (MUSCULAR)

PSAX-PML

INLET VSDs (MUSCULAR)
- Infracristal
- Supracristal

BE Bulwer, MD

Base of Heart
(atria removed)

Outlet VSDs
Supracristal
Infracristal
Membranous VSDs
Inlet VSDs
Inlet - Atrioventricular canal type VSDs

Quantification of VSD shunt
Qp:Qs

$$\frac{\pi(RVOT\ radius)^2 \times VTI_{RVOT}}{\pi(LVOT\ radius)^2 \times VTI_{LVOT}}$$

PSAX -AVL

Outlet VSDs
Supracristal ~1 - 2 o'clock
Infracristal ~12 o'clock
Membranous, Perimembranous VSDs ~10 - 11 o'clock
Septal leaflet of tricuspid valve (TV)

Progressive Right heart dilatation, hypertrophy, tricuspid regurgitation

VSD shunt

Pulmonary artery (PA) dilatation
RV hypertrophy

Shunt reversal; cyanosis

Restrictive VSD	Moderately restrictive VSD	Non-restrictive VSD	Eisenmenger VSD
Qp/Qs: < 1.4	Qp/Qs: 1.4 - 2.2	Qp/Qs: > 2.2	Qp/Qs: < 1.1
PASP/AP: < 0.3	PASP/AP: > 0.3 < 0.66	PASP/AP: > 0.66	PASP/AP: 1.0

AP: aortic presssure; PASP: pulmonary artery systolic pressure; Qp: pulmonary flow (cardiac output); Qs: systemic flow (cardiac output); Qp:Qs - Pulmonary: Systemic flow ratio, RVOT/LVOT: right/left ventricular outflow tract, VTI: velocity time integral measured by PW Doppler

RIGHT VENTRICULAR (RV) INFLOW VIEW

The RV inflow view focuses on examination of the structure and function of the right heart chambers, including the tricuspid valve.

Patient and transducer positioning

Patient remains in the left lateral decubitus position, unchanged from the PLAX view Figure 6.35 .

Transducer maneuvers

From the PLAX position, slightly angulate the transducer toward the right hip using the maneuver shown in Figure 6.35 , and adjust the scan plane to focus on the tricuspid valve until the structures shown in Figure 6.39 are optimally visualized. Avoid inclusion of the LV and other left-sided structures. The RV inflow view is one that most novice sonographers find especially challenging.

Transducer scan plane orientation and anatomy

As is evident from Figures 6.35–6.38 , the transducer scan plane sweeps across and away from the aortic root and left-sided structures, including the LV and the interventricular septum (IVS), and toward the right atrium (RA), tricuspid valve (TV), and right ventricle (RV).

2D scan sector image display

Identify, optimize, and record the structures shown in Figures 6.37–6.39 . As this view is the least standardized view of the transthoracic examination, some acceptable variations can be recorded. The large anterior TV leaflet is seen in almost all views of the TV (with its insertion into the free wall of the RV) along with either the septal or inferoposterior leaflet. When the inferoposterior leaflet of the TV is recorded (instead of the IVS and the septal leaflet), the inferior wall, as it receives the coronary sinus (CS) and the inferior vena cava (IVC), is easily seen Figures 6.37–6.40 . When the septal leaflet of the TV is recorded along with its insertions in the IVS, a portion of the LV cavity is seen (Figure 6.40 , bottom right panel).

Color flow Doppler exam

Apply color Doppler, and position color scan sector over the TV, IVC, and CS and examine color flow patterns. Note the Doppler alignment results in red flow velocities moving from RA to RV across the TV and toward the transducer Figure 6.40 . Tricuspid regurgitation (TR), present to a mild degree in most (~75%) normal individuals, would appear as blue flow velocities away from the transducer Figures 4.13, 6.43 . Confirm the presence and the extent of the TR jet when examining the tricuspid valve on the subsequent views: PSAX-AVL, A4C, SC-4C.

Spectral (CW) Doppler exam

Because of the Doppler alignment, the spectral Doppler display of the RV inflow velocities appears above the baseline, whereas TR velocities—which are directed away from the transducer—appear below the baseline Figure 6.41 . Corroborate the findings of TR on subsequent views—specifically on the PSAX-AVL and A4C views—and assess peak TR velocities Figure 6.43 . Analysis of the CW Doppler velocity profile provides important information on right heart hemodynamics. When used in conjunction with other echocardiographic and Doppler parameters, right-side pressures—corresponding to those obtained on cardiac catheterization—can be quantified. Such parameters include visual assessment of IVC behavior, PW and CW Doppler to the pulmonary valve (PV), PW Doppler of mitral valve (MV) inflow, and tissue Doppler assessment of the mitral annular velocities Figures 4.5, 6.42 .

Findings and Summaries

Assess cardiac structure and function. Confirm normal and abnormal findings on complementary views Table 6.2 ; Figures 6.43, 6.44 .

RIGHT VENTRICULAR (RV) INFLOW VIEW: PATIENT POSITIONING, TRANSDUCER PLACEMENT, AND SCAN PLANE

Optimize the view and acquire at depths of 20 and 15–16 cm. Evaluate the tricuspid valve (by zooming or decrease depth). Apply color Doppler Figure 6.40 , and follow up by continuous-wave (CW) Doppler interrogation of flow across the tricuspid valve Figure 6.41 .

Figure 6.35

Patient and transducer positioning: RV inflow view.

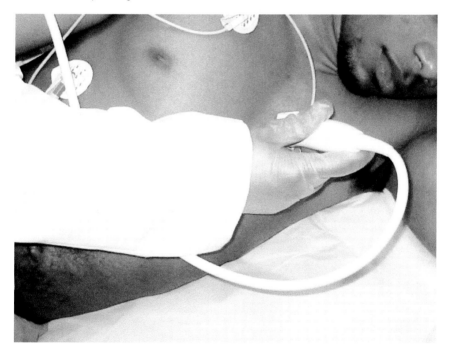

After recording the PLAX view, the patient's position and transducer index mark orientation remain largely unchanged. Slightly angulate the transducer toward the right hip until the RV inflow view comes into focus Figures 6.36–6.40 .

Figure 6.36

Right ventricle inflow scan plane.

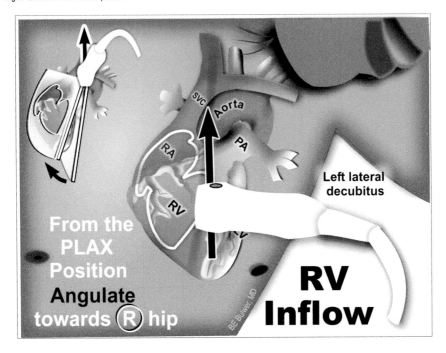

From the PLAX scan plane, slightly angulate the transducer scan plane medially and slightly inferiorly toward the right hip. Additionally, mild degrees of rotation, ~15° to 30° clockwise or anticlockwise, may be necessary to optimally visualize the RV inflow view.

RV INFLOW VIEW: SCAN PLANE, ANATOMY, AND SCAN SECTOR DISPLAY
Figure 6.37

Panoramic perspectives of the RV inflow scan plane, scan plane anatomy, and image display. When properly acquired, the RV inflow scan plane transects the major cardiac structures shown. *Upper-left and mid-left panels*. Angulation of the transducer results in a sweep away from the left side of the heart and toward the right side. This means that the RV inflow scan plane "slices" a "chip" off the right heart, as shown in the anatomical views (see Figures 6.2–6.5). *Bottom*. The RV inflow scan plane anatomy that corresponds to the image display is better appreciated if viewed from the right side of the supine patient. This puts the right ventricle (RV) above the right atrium (RA), from the viewpoint of the transducer. *Upper-right and mid-right panels*. On the image display, blood flows upward (toward the transducer) from the RA via the tricuspid valve (TV) into the RV. Therefore, the Doppler flow velocities on the RV inflow view appear red, with spectral profiles above the baseline. For the same reason, the jet of tricuspid regurgitation (TR), where flow velocities are directed away from the transducer, appear blue, with spectral Doppler profiles displayed below the baseline (Figures 6.40, 6.41).

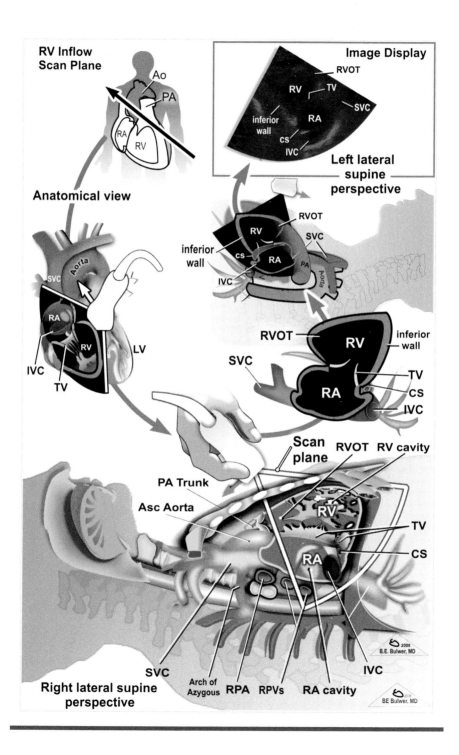

RV Inflow
Scan Plane

Ao

PA

RA

RV

Anatomical view

Image Display

RVOT

RV — TV

SVC

inferior
wall

RA

cs

IVC

Left lateral
supine
perspective

Aorta

SVC

RA

RV

LV

IVC

TV

RVOT

inferior
wall

cs

RA

PA

IVC

Aorta

RVOT

RV

inferior
wall

SVC

TV

RA

cs

IVC

Scan
plane

RVOT RV cavity

PA Trunk

Asc Aorta

RV

TV

cs

RA

SVC

IVC

Right lateral supine
perspective

Arch of
Azygous RPA RPVs RA cavity

2008
B.E. Bulwer, MD

2008
BE Bulwer, MD

RV INFLOW VIEW: SCAN PLANE ANATOMY
Figure 6.38

The RV inflow scan plane and the major anatomical structures transected.

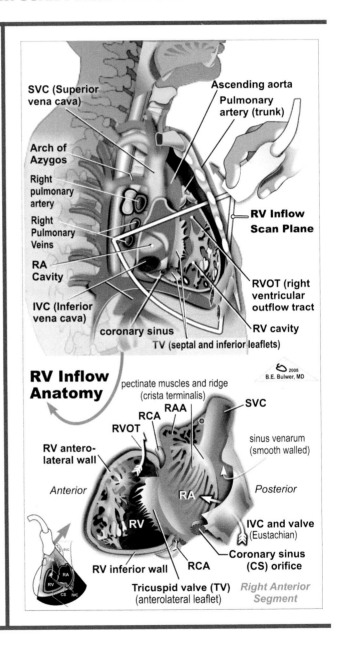

SVC (Superior vena cava)

Ascending aorta

Pulmonary artery (trunk)

Arch of Azygos

Right pulmonary artery

Right Pulmonary Veins

RA Cavity

IVC (Inferior vena cava)

coronary sinus

TV (septal and inferior leaflets)

RV Inflow Scan Plane

RVOT (right ventricular outflow tract

RV cavity

RV Inflow Anatomy

pectinate muscles and ridge (crista terminalis)

RAA

RCA

RVOT

RV antero-lateral wall

Anterior

SVC

sinus venarum (smooth walled)

Posterior

RA

RV

RV inferior wall

RCA

Tricuspid valve (TV) (anterolateral leaflet)

IVC and valve (Eustachian)

Coronary sinus (CS) orifice

Right Anterior Segment

2008
B.E. Bulwer, MD

RV INFLOW VIEW: SCAN SECTOR ANATOMY AND COLOR FLOW DOPPLER EXAMINATION
Figure 6.39

Right ventricular inflow view. Optimally assess and record structures shown.

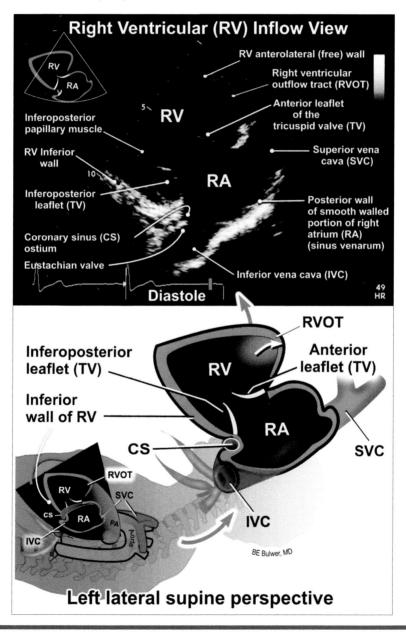

Figure 6.40

Right ventricular inflow view showing flow schema and color flow velocities. Compare with Figure 6.37 and legend.

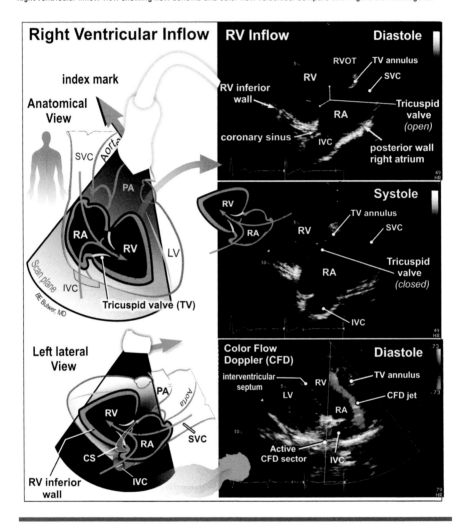

RV INFLOW VIEW: CONTINUOUS-WAVE (CW) DOPPLER EXAMINATION OF THE TRICUSPID VALVE

Figure 6.41

Right ventricular (RV) inflow and outflow. Color Doppler-guided CW Doppler examination of the tricuspid valve.

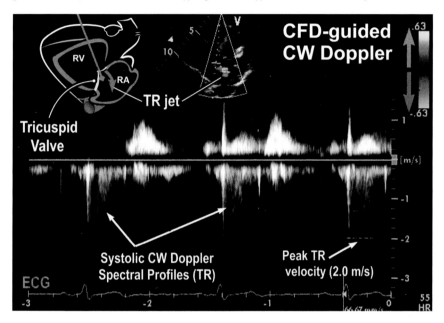

At each step of the transthoracic examination, the color flow Doppler examination precedes the spectral (PW, CW) Doppler examination. Color flow Doppler serves as an important map or guide for optimal placement and alignment of the spectral Doppler sample volume.

To assess flow velocities across the tricuspid valve, optimally align and position the PW Doppler sample volume at the tips of the tricuspid leaflets. This normally reveals an upward biphasic spectral Doppler profile of RV inflow, which is akin to that of the LV transmitral inflow, but this is better appreciated from the PSAX-AVL and A4C views Figures 6.55, 7.14–7.16 .

The flow of tricuspid regurgitation (TR) moves in the opposite direction, with flow velocities directed away from the transducer. This appears as blue flow velocities on the color flow Doppler examination, with TR velocity profiles appearing below the baseline on spectral Doppler. Tricuspid regurgitation is a normal finding in up to 75% of normal individuals.

Peak TR velocities on CW Doppler, as shown in Figure 6.41 , measured 2.0 m/s. This can be converted into pressure gradients (driving pressure) using the simplified Bernoulli equation: $P = 4v^2$ Figure 4.14 . In this instance, this translates into a pulmonary artery systolic pressure (PASP) of $4(2)^2$ mmHg or 16 mmHg plus the right atrial pressure (RAP) Figures 4.5, 6.42 . The latter is estimated from observing the respirophasic behavior (or degree of inspiratory collapse) of the inferior vena cava when observed on the subcostal examination of the IVC (SC-IVC).

"ECHO RIGHT-HEART CATHETERIZATION"
Figure 6.42

Echocardiographic correlates of right heart catheterization.

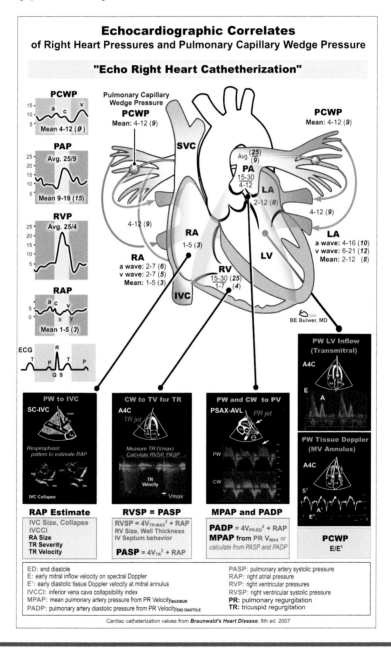

Echocardiographic Correlates of Right Heart Pressures and Pulmonary Capillary Wedge Pressure. "Echo Right Heart Cathetherization"

ED: end diastole
E: early mitral inflow velocity on spectral Doppler
E': early diastolic tissue Doppler velocity at mitral annulus
IVCCI: inferior vena cava collapsibility index
MPAP: mean pulmonary artery pressure from PR Velocity_MAXIMUM
PADP: pulmonary artery diastolic pressure from PR Velocity_END DIASTOLE

PASP: pulmonary artery systolic pressure
RAP: right atrial pressure
RVP: right ventricular pressures
RVSP: right ventricular systolic pressure
PR: pulmonary regurgitation
TR: tricuspid regurgitation

Cardiac catheterization values from *Braunwald's Heart Disease*, 8th ed. 2007

Table 6.2 RIGHT VENTRICULAR (RV)INFLOW VIEW: THE EXAMINATION SURVEY

Sequential survey (by flow sequence)	RV Inflow View	
	Structural: on 2D, 3D, or M-mode	Functional and hemodynamic (on Doppler, including color Doppler)
Right atrium (RA)	RA CAVITY SIZE [Fig. 6.44] • Size: Normal, increased, decreased • RA enlargement: mild, moderate, severe: (note post cardiac transplant, cor triatriatum) RA CAVITY APPEARANCE • Mass—most commonly thrombus (clot), myxoma • Mass—Chiari network • Cardiac hardware: pacer or defibrillator wire, catheter (Swan Ganz) • "Smoke" (spontaneous echocontrast) • RA dimensions RA VIEWS • See [Fig. 6.44]	RA PHASIC DYNAMICS • RA acts as "reservoir-conduit-pump" • Loss of atrial "pump" (**atrial fibrillation**) • Diastolic collapse of RA free wall—earliest sign in **pericardial tamponade** [Fig. 6.33] RA PRESSURES (RAP) [Figs. 4.5, 6.42] **Signs of elevated RAP** • Dilated IVC with decreased respirophasic collapse—use subcostal-IVC view (see [Fig. 8.9b] ; [Table 8.1]) • Dilated tributary veins: IVC, SVC, coronary sinus • Dilated RA, RV • Severe TR • Bowing of interatrial septum toward the left (thoughout cardiac cycle)
Tricuspid valve (TV)	TV STRUCTURE • **Normal leaflet structure, mobility, thickness, and closure:** (coaptation), chordae tendinae, papillary muscle • **Leaflet vegetation:** location, size, mobility TV LEAFLET MOBILITY • **Excessive movement of one or both leaflets:** prolapse, leaflet flail • **Restricted leaflet motion:** thickened immobile leaflets in carcinoid syndrome, rheumatic fever (rare) • Prosthetic TV: mechanical vs. bioprosthetic; normal vs. abnormal function; valve and paravalvular dysfunction	TRICUSPID REGURGITATION (TR) • Peak velocity: CW Doppler • PASP (pulmonary artery systolic pressure) measurement (applying the Bernoulli equation to peak CW Doppler velocities). Add to right atrial pressure (RAP) estimates from IVC assessment (subcostal IVC view) [Figs. 4.5, 6.40–6.42] • Assess etiology • Estimate severity: mild, moderate, severe [Fig. 6.43a] TRICUSPID STENOSIS (TS) • Assess etiology (carcinoid, rheumatic) • Estimate severity: mild, moderate, severe [Fig. 6.43b]

Table 6.2 RIGHT VENTRICULAR (RV)INFLOW VIEW:
THE EXAMINATION SURVEY *(continued)*

Sequential survey (by flow sequence)	RV Inflow View	
	Structural: on 2D, 3D, or M-mode	Functional and hemodynamic (on Doppler, including color Doppler)
Right ventricle (RV)	RV CAVITY SIZE Figs. 6.31, 6.32 ; Table 12.5 • Size: normal, increased, or decreased • RV dilatation in RV pressure and volume overload states, e.g., right heart failure; primary and secondary pulmonary hypertension; secundum ASD Fig. 6.44 RV/RVOT FREE WALL • Thickened in chronic overload states, e.g., chronic pulmonary hypertension RV MASSES • Thromboembolus (clot) • Tumor • Cardiac hardware, e.g., pacemaker, defibrillator wire, Swan Ganz catheter—traverses tricuspid valve	RV SYSTOLIC FUNCTION Fig. 6.32 (As for PLAX view; see Table 6.1) • Impaired contractility in RV pressure and volume overload states • Systolic dysfunction (confirm with other views of RV) RV FREE WALL • Diastolic collapse with pericardial tamponade • RVOT diastolic collapse consistent with tamponade physiology; confirm on other views and M-mode Fig. 6.33
Inferior vena cava (IVC) and eustachian valve	• Dilated IVC (see Fig. 8.9b ; Table 8.1) • Eustachian valve vs. thrombus • Chiari network (sinus venosum remnant—nonpathologic): differentiate from mobile thromboembolus	• Respirophasic behavior (IVC collapsibility index; Figs. 4.5, 6.42 ; Table 8.1) • Flow reversal into IVC and hepatic veins (color flow Doppler) in severe tricuspid regurgitation (TR) Fig. 6.43a
Coronary Sinus (CS)	• Dilated chamber—if marked, consider persistent L superior vena cava (PLSVC) • Cardiac hardware, e.g., defibrillator wire; MV support device to treat MR	• Confirm PLSVC by agitated saline "bubble" study injected into L arm vein. This opacifies coronary sinus before it enters RA.

TRICUSPID REGURGITATION
Figure 6.43a

Echocardiographic assessment of tricuspid regurgitation: a summary.

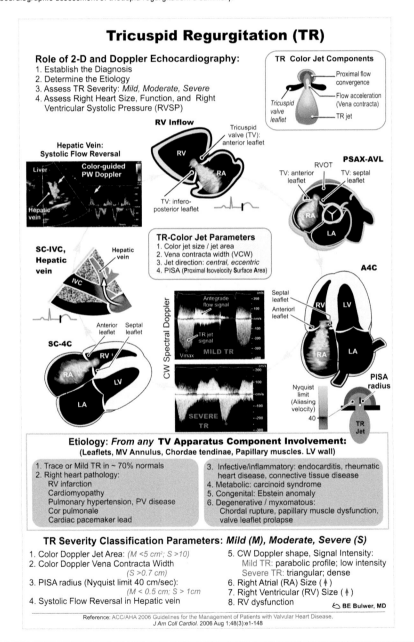

Tricuspid Regurgitation (TR)

Role of 2-D and Doppler Echocardiography:
1. Establish the Diagnosis
2. Determine the Etiology
3. Assess TR Severity: *Mild, Moderate, Severe*
4. Assess Right Heart Size, Function, and Right Ventricular Systolic Pressure (RVSP)

TR Color Jet Components
- Proximal flow convergence
- Flow acceleration (Vena contracta)
- TR jet

RV Inflow

Hepatic Vein: Systolic Flow Reversal
Color-guided PW Doppler

SC-IVC, Hepatic vein

SC-4C

TR-Color Jet Parameters
1. Color jet size / jet area
2. Vena contracta width (VCW)
3. Jet direction: *central, eccentric*
4. PISA (Proximal Isovelocity Surface Area)

PSAX-AVL

A4C

CW Spectral Doppler — MILD TR — SEVERE TR

PISA radius
Nyquist limit (Aliasing velocity) 40

Etiology: *From any* TV Apparatus Component Involvement:
(Leaflets, MV Annulus, Chordae tendinae, Papillary muscles. LV wall)

1. Trace or Mild TR in ~ 70% normals
2. Right heart pathology:
   RV infarction
   Cardiomyopathy
   Pulmonary hypertension, PV disease
   Cor pulmonale
   Cardiac pacemaker lead
3. Infective/inflammatory: endocarditis, rheumatic heart disease, connective tissue disease
4. Metabolic: carcinoid syndrome
5. Congenital: Ebstein anomaly
6. Degenerative / myxomatous:
   Chordal rupture, papillary muscle dysfunction, valve leaflet prolapse

TR Severity Classification Parameters: *Mild (M), Moderate, Severe (S)*

1. Color Doppler Jet Area: *(M <5 cm²; S >10)*
2. Color Doppler Vena Contracta Width *(S >0.7 cm)*
3. PISA radius (Nyquist limit 40 cm/sec): *(M < 0.5 cm; S > 1cm)*
4. Systolic Flow Reversal in Hepatic vein
5. CW Doppler shape, Signal Intensity:
   Mild TR: parabolic profile; low intensity
   Severe TR: triangular; dense
6. Right Atrial (RA) Size (↕)
7. Right Ventricular (RV) Size (↕)
8. RV dysfunction

BE Bulwer, MD

Reference: ACC/AHA 2006 Guidelines for the Management of Patients with Valvular Heart Disease.
J Am Coll Cardiol. 2006 Aug 1;48(3):e1-148

TRICUSPID STENOSIS
Figure 6.43b

Echocardiographic assessment of mitral stenosis: a summary.

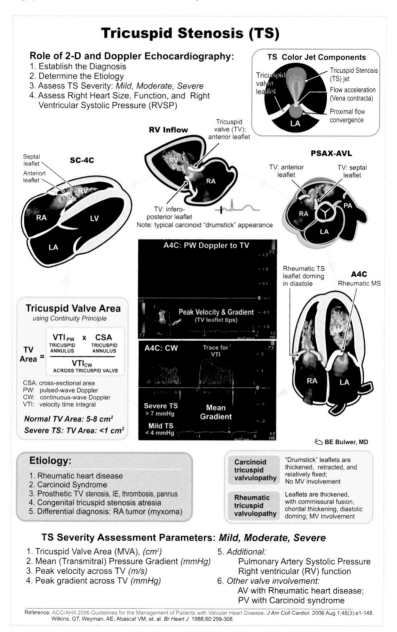

Tricuspid Stenosis (TS)

Role of 2-D and Doppler Echocardiography:
1. Establish the Diagnosis
2. Determine the Etiology
3. Assess TS Severity: *Mild, Moderate, Severe*
4. Assess Right Heart Size, Function, and Right Ventricular Systolic Pressure (RVSP)

TS Color Jet Components
- Tricuspid Stenosis (TS) jet
- Flow acceleration (Vena contracta)
- Proximal flow convergence
- Tricuspid valve leaflet
- LA

RV Inflow
Tricuspid valve (TV): anterior leaflet

SC-4C
- Septal leaflet
- Anteriorl leaflet
- RV

TV: infero-posterior leaflet
Note: typical carcinoid "drumstick" appearance

PSAX-AVL
- TV: anterior leaflet
- TV: septal leaflet
- RA
- PA
- LA

A4C: PW Doppler to TV

Peak Velocity & Gradient (TV leaflet tips)

A4C: CW — Trace for VTI

Rheumatic TS leaflet doming in diastole

A4C Rheumatic MS

Severe TS > 7 mmHg
Mild TS < 4 mmHg

Mean Gradient

Tricuspid Valve Area
using Continuity Principle

$$\text{TV Area} = \frac{VTI_{PW}\ _{TRICUSPID\ ANNULUS} \times CSA\ _{TRICUSPID\ ANNULUS}}{VTI_{CW}\ _{ACROSS\ TRICUSPID\ VALVE}}$$

CSA: cross-sectional area
PW: pulsed-wave Doppler
CW: continuous-wave Doppler
VTI: velocity time integral

Normal TV Area: 5-8 cm²
Severe TS: TV Area: <1 cm²

✍ BE Bulwer, MD

Etiology:
1. Rheumatic heart disease
2. Carcinoid Syndrome
3. Prosthetic TV stenosis, IE, thrombosis, pannus
4. Congenital tricuspid stenosis atresia
5. Differential diagnosis: RA tumor (myxoma)

Carcinoid tricuspid valvulopathy: "Drumstick" leaflets are thickened, retracted, and relatively fixed; No MV involvement

Rheumatic tricuspid valvulopathy: Leaflets are thickened, with commissural fusion, chordal thickening, diastolic doming; MV involvement

TS Severity Assessment Parameters: *Mild, Moderate, Severe*
1. Tricuspid Valve Area (MVA), *(cm²)*
2. Mean (Transmitral) Pressure Gradient *(mmHg)*
3. Peak velocity across TV *(m/s)*
4. Peak gradient across TV *(mmHg)*
5. *Additional:*
   Pulmonary Artery Systolic Pressure
   Right ventricular (RV) function
6. *Other valve involvement:*
   AV with Rheumatic heart disease;
   PV with Carcinoid syndrome

Reference: ACC/AHA 2006 Guidelines for the Management of Patients with Valvular Heart Disease. *J Am Coll Cardiol.* 2006 Aug 1;48(3):e1-148. Wilkins, GT, Weyman, AE, Abascal VM, et. al. *Br Heart J* 1988;60:299-308.

RIGHT ATRIUM
Figure 6.44

Echocardiographic assessment of the right atrium.

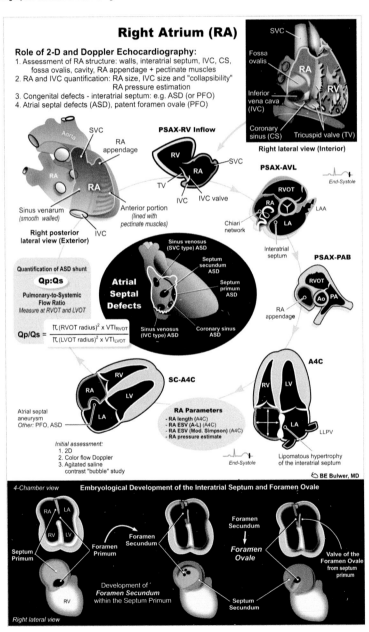

Right Atrium (RA)

Role of 2-D and Doppler Echocardiography:
1. Assessment of RA structure: walls, interatrial septum, IVC, CS, fossa ovalis, cavity, RA appendage + pectinate muscles
2. RA and IVC quantification: RA size, IVC size and "collapsibility" RA pressure estimation
3. Congenital defects - interatrial septum: e.g. ASD (or PFO)
4. Atrial septal defects (ASD), patent foramen ovale (PFO)

Right lateral view (Interior)

Right posterior lateral view (Exterior)

PSAX-RV Inflow

PSAX-AVL

PSAX-PAB

Atrial Septal Defects
- Sinus venosus (SVC type) ASD
- Septum secundum ASD
- Septum primum ASD
- Sinus venosus (IVC type) ASD
- Coronary sinus ASD

Quantification of ASD shunt

Qp:Qs

Pulmonary-to-Systemic Flow Ratio
Measure at RVOT and LVOT

$$Qp/Qs = \frac{\pi(RVOT\ radius)^2 \times VTI_{RVOT}}{\pi(LVOT\ radius)^2 \times VTI_{LVOT}}$$

SC-A4C

Atrial septal aneurysm
Other: PFO, ASD

RA Parameters
- RA length (A4C)
- RA ESV (A-L) (A4C)
- RA ESV (Mod. Simpson) (A4C)
- RA pressure estimate

Initial assessment:
1. 2D
2. Color flow Doppler
3. Agitated saline contrast "bubble" study

A4C

Lipomatous hypertrophy of the interatrial septum

⟨◎⟩ BE Bulwer, MD

Embryological Development of the Interatrial Septum and Foramen Ovale

4-Chamber view

Foramen Secundum

Foramen Ovale

Septum Primum

Foramen Primum

Foramen Secundum

Development of *Foramen Secundum* within the Septum Primum

Septum Secundum

Valve of the Foramen Ovale from septum primum

Right lateral view

RIGHT VENTRICULAR (RV) OUTFLOW VIEW

The RV outflow view is used to assess the right ventricular outflow tract (RVOT), the main pulmonary artery (PA), and the intervening pulmonary valve (PV).

Patient and transducer positioning

Patient remains in the left lateral decubitus position, as with the PLAX and RV inflow views Figure 6.45 .

Transducer maneuvers

From the RV inflow position, angulate the transducer toward the left shoulder, using the maneuver of the transducer scan plane as shown in Figures 6.45, 6.46 . This sweeps the scan plane from the right-sided structures to the left-sided structures, and unto the RVOT, PV, and PA. This usually requires slight degrees of clockwise rotation to bring these structures into focus. Optimize the view Figures 6.46, 6.47a .

Transducer scan plane orientation and anatomy

The transducer scan plane transects the RV outflow tract and pulmonary artery, as shown in Figures 6.46 and 6.47 . Note the crescentic RVOT as it arches around the LV, separated from the main pulmonary artery by the pulmonary valve. On the RV outflow view, the bifurcation of the main pulmonary trunk is not usually seen.

2D scan sector image display

Identify, optimize, and record the landmark structures: RV outflow tract, pulmonary valve (PV), and main pulmonary artery Figures 6.46, 6.47 .

Color flow Doppler exam

Apply color Doppler to the RV outflow tract, pulmonary valve, and the main pulmonary artery (trunk). Note that the Doppler alignment results in blue flow velocities moving from RVOT to PA, i.e., away from the transducer Figure 6.47b . Pulmonary regurgitation is a common finding in normal individuals, and it would appear as diastolic red flow velocities toward the transducer Figure 6.48a . RVOT obstruction and pulmonary artery stenosis exhibit flow acceleration patterns distal to the site of obstruction or stenosis Figure 6.48b .

Spectral (PW, CW) Doppler exam

The normal spectral Doppler interrogation of the pulmonary valve shows flow velocities appearing below the baseline. This represents blood flow away from the transducer Figure 6.48a . Corroborate the findings of PR and TR on subsequent views, specifically on the PSAX-AVL and A4C views, and assess peak PR and TR velocities Figure 6.48a . From this, important information on right heart hemodynamics, in conjunction with other parameters of right-side pressures, can be quantified Figures 4.5, 6.42 .

Findings and Summaries

Assess cardiac structure and function. Confirm normal and abnormal findings using subsequent views Table 6.2 ; Figures 6.48a, 6.48b .

RV OUTFLOW VIEW: PATIENT POSITIONING, TRANSDUCER PLACEMENT, AND SCAN PLANE

The sonographer may opt to image the RV outflow by angling superolaterally with the transducer scan plane that transects the pulmonary artery (PA), as shown in Figures 6.45–6.47 . This is followed by Doppler evaluation of the pulmonary valves Figures 6.47–6.48 .

This view provides good visualization of the pulmonary valves and the bifurcation of the main PA trunk into the right and left pulmonary arteries—sometimes called the "trunk and trousers" view. Note that anatomically, it is the right pulmonary artery that is directly related to the ascending portion of the aorta anteriorly.

Figure 6.45

Right ventricular (RV) outflow scan plane. From the RV inflow position, angulate the scan plane toward the left shoulder, with slight degree of rotation to optimize the structures of interest: the right ventricular outflow tract (RVOT), the pulmonary valve (PV), and the main pulmonary artery (PA).

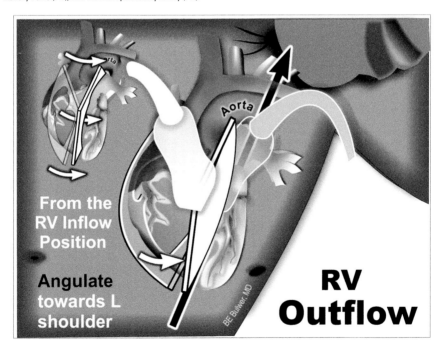

RV OUTFLOW VIEW: SCAN PLANE, ANATOMY, AND SCAN SECTOR DISPLAY

Figure 6.46

Panoramic perspectives of the RV outflow scan plane, scan plane anatomy, and image display. When properly acquired, the RV outflow scan plane transects the major cardiac structures shown. *Upper-left and mid-left panels.* Angulation away from the RV inflow view scan plane and toward the left shoulder brings into focus the RV outflow tract (RVOT) scan plane (see Figures 6.2–6.5). Mild clockwise rotation is often needed to visualize the long-axis of the main pulmonary artery (PA) and the intervening pulmonary valve (PV). *Bottom.* When viewed from the left lateral supine perspective, blood flow from the RVOT to the PA is directed away from the transducer. *Upper-right and mid-right panels.* On the image display, blood flows downward (away from the transducer) from the RVOT via the pulmonary valve (PV) and into the PA. Therefore, the Doppler flow velocities on the RV outflow view appear blue (Figure 6.47b), with spectral profiles below the baseline (Figure 6.48a).

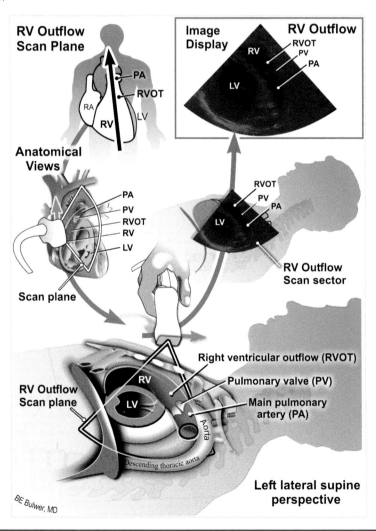

RV OUTFLOW VIEW: SCAN PLANE AND SCAN SECTOR ANATOMY

Figure 6.47a

RV outflow scan plane, scan plane anatomy, and image display. *LV: left ventricle; PA: main pulmonary artery (pulmonary trunk); PV: pulmonary valve; RV: right ventricle; RVOT: right ventricular outflow tract.*

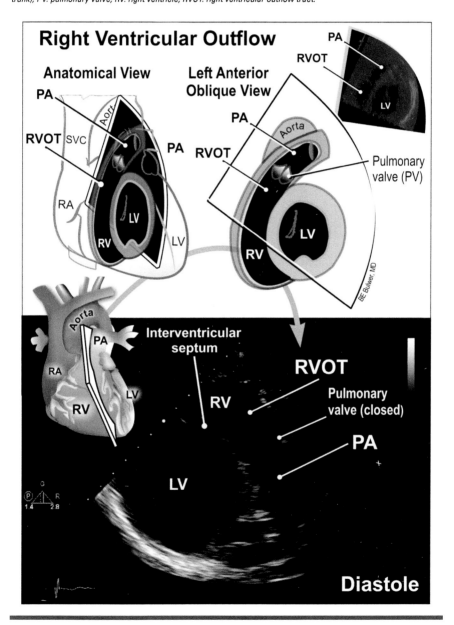

RV OUTFLOW VIEW: COLOR FLOW DOPPLER EXAMINATION
Figure 6.47b

Right ventricular (RV) outflow tract: perspectives on blood flow patterns and color flow Doppler display. Note that flow within the RV outflow tract and pulmonary artery is directed away from the transducer; therefore, blue color velocities on color flow Doppler and spectral Doppler velocity profiles below the baseline. The diastolic jet of pulmonary regurgitant appears red, with spectral Doppler profiles displayed above the baseline (Figure 6.48a).

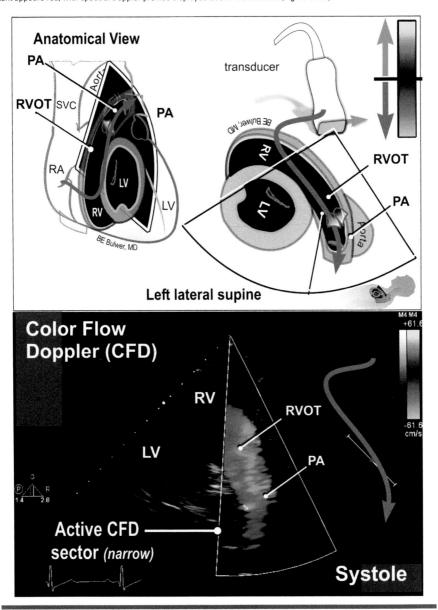

RV OUTFLOW SURVEY: NORMAL AND ABNORMAL FINDINGS

Table 6.3 RIGHT VENTRICULAR (RV) OUTFLOW VIEW: THE EXAMINATION SURVEY

Sequential survey	Findings: RV outflow-pulmonary artery view	
	Structural: on 2D, 3D, or M-mode	Functional and hemodynamic (on Doppler, including color Doppler)
Right ventricle (RV) and right ventricular outflow tract (RVOT)	RVOT CAVITY SIZE ⟨Figs. 6.31 and 6.32⟩ ; ⟨Table 12.5⟩ • RV dilatation in RV pressure and volume overload states RV/ RVOT FREE WALL • Thickened in chronic overload states, e.g., chronic pulmonary hypertension RV MASSES • Cardiac hardware, e.g., Swan-Ganz catheter—traverses tricuspid valve	RV SYSTOLIC FUNCTION ⟨Fig. 6.32⟩ • Impaired contractility in RV pressure and volume overload states RV FREE WALL • Diastolic collapse with pericardial tamponade • RVOT diastolic collapse consistent with tamponade physiology; confirm on other views and M-mode ⟨Fig. 6.33⟩
Pulmonary valve (PV)	PV STRUCTURE • Observe normally trileaflet (cusps) structure and annulus • Thickened immobile leaflets in carcinoid syndrome • Pulmonary stenosis (PS) • Thromboemboli • Pulmonary band or residual from previous interventions in congenital heart disease	PULMONARY REGURGITATION (PR) • Assess etiology • Estimate severity: mild, moderate, severe ⟨Fig. 6.48a⟩ PULMONARY STENOSIS (PS) • Assess etiology • Estimate severity: mild, moderate, severe ⟨Fig. 6.48b⟩
Pulmonary artery (PA)	• Dilatation • Stenosis • Embolus ± saddle embolus at bifurcation • Cardiac hardware, e.g., Swan-Ganz catheter • Pulmonary artery dimensions ⟨Fig. 6.48a⟩ ; ⟨Table 12.5⟩	• PW and CW evidence of pulmonary stenosis, regurgitation • Estimates of pulmonary artery pressures (echocardiographic correlates of right heart catheterization; ⟨Figs. 4.5, 6.42, 8.10⟩ ; ⟨Table 8.1⟩

PULMONARY REGURGITATION

The RV outflow view is used to assess the right ventricular outflow tract (RVOT), the main pulmonary artery (PA), and the intervening pulmonary valve (PV).

Figure 6.48a

Echocardiographic assessment of pulmonary regurgitation: a summary.

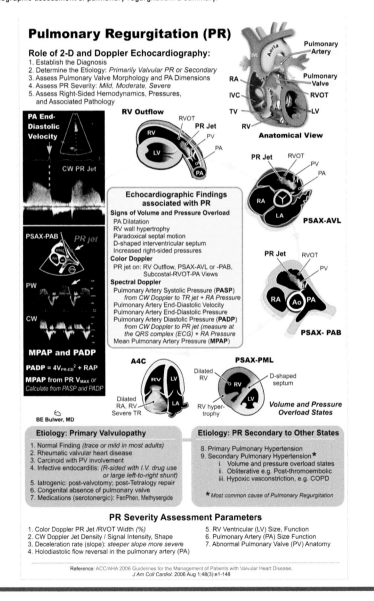

Pulmonary Regurgitation (PR)

Role of 2-D and Doppler Echocardiography:
1. Establish the Diagnosis
2. Determine the Etiology: *Primarily Valvular PR or Secondary*
3. Assess Pulmonary Valve Morphology and PA Dimensions
4. Assess PR Severity: *Mild, Moderate, Severe*
5. Assess Right-Sided Hemodynamics, Pressures, and Associated Pathology

Anatomical View

Echocardiographic Findings associated with PR

Signs of Volume and Pressure Overload
PA Dilatation
RV wall hypertrophy
Paradoxical septal motion
D-shaped interventricular septum
Increased right-sided pressures

Color Doppler
PR jet on: RV Outflow, PSAX-AVL or -PAB, Subcostal-RVOT-PA Views

Spectral Doppler
Pulmonary Artery Systolic Pressure (**PASP**)
  from CW Doppler to TR jet + RA Pressure
Pulmonary Artery End-Diastolic Velocity
Pulmonary Artery End-Diastolic Pressure
Pulmonary Artery Diastolic Pressure (**PADP**)
  from CW Doppler to PR jet (measure at the QRS complex (ECG) + RA Pressure
Mean Pulmonary Artery Pressure (**MPAP**)

MPAP and PADP

$PADP = 4V_{PR-ED}^2 + RAP$

MPAP from PR V_{MAX} *or*
Calculate from PASP and PADP

BE Bulwer, MD

Volume and Pressure Overload States

Etiology: Primary Valvulopathy
1. Normal Finding *(trace or mild in most adults)*
2. Rheumatic valvular heart disease
3. Carcinoid with PV involvement
4. Infective endocarditis: *(R-sided with I.V. drug use or large left-to-right shunt)*
5. Iatrogenic: post-valvotomy; post-Tetralogy repair
6. Congenital absence of pulmonary valve
7. Medications (serotonergic): FenPhen, Methysergide

Etiology: PR Secondary to Other States
8. Primary Pulmonary Hypertension
9. Secondary Pulmonary Hypertension*
  i. Volume and pressure overload states
  ii. Obliterative e.g. Post-thromoembolic
  iii. Hypoxic vasconstriction, e.g. COPD

★ Most common cause of Pulmonary Regurgitation

PR Severity Assessment Parameters
1. Color Doppler PR Jet /RVOT Width *(%)*
2. CW Doppler Jet Density / Signal Intensity, Shape
3. Deceleration rate (slope): *steeper slope more severe*
4. Holodiastolic flow reversal in the pulmonary artery (PA)
5. RV Ventricular (LV) Size, Function
6. Pulmonary Artery (PA) Size Function
7. Abnormal Pulmonary Valve (PV) Anatomy

Reference: ACC/AHA 2006 Guidelines for the Management of Patients with Valvular Heart Disease.
J Am Coll Cardiol. 2006 Aug 1;48(3):e1-148

PULMONARY STENOSIS

The RV outflow view is used to assess the right ventricular outflow tract (RVOT), the main pulmonary artery (PA), and the intervening pulmonary valve (PV).

Figure 6.48b

Echocardiographic assessment of pulmonary stenosis: a summary.

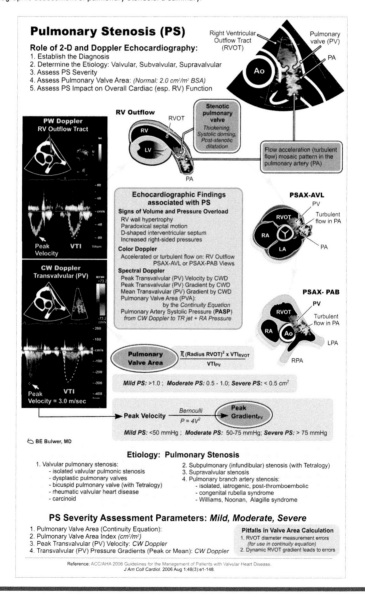

LEFT PARASTERNAL SHORT-AXIS VIEW: SCAN PLANES
Figure 6.49

A family of parasternal short-axis (PSAX) scan planes as viewed from both the anatomical position and with the patient in the left lateral decubitus position (see Figure 6.50).

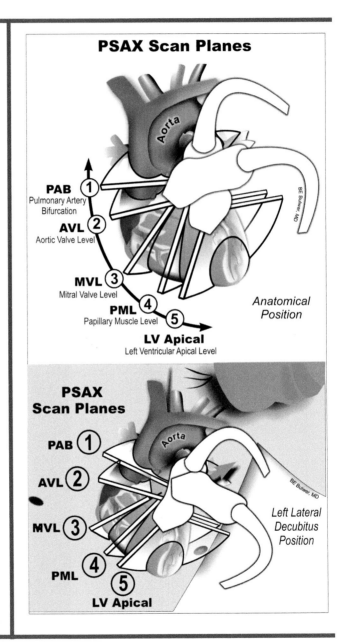

PSAX Scan Planes

BE Bulwer, MD

PAB ① Pulmonary Artery Bifurcation

AVL ② Aortic Valve Level

MVL ③ Mitral Valve Level

PML ④ Papillary Muscle Level ⑤

LV Apical Left Ventricular Apical Level

Anatomical Position

PSAX Scan Planes

PAB ①

AVL ②

MVL ③

PML ④ ⑤

LV Apical

Left Lateral Decubitus Position

BE Bulwer, MD

PSAX SCAN PLANES, VIEWS, AND SCAN SECTOR DISPLAY
Figure 6.50

Parasternal short-axis (PSAX) family of scan planes, scan plane anatomy, and scan sector image displays. Note the cross-sectional anatomy and the corresponding image displays that result when the scan plane sweeps from the base of the heart superiorly toward the apex inferiorly, i.e., through scan planes 1→2→3→4→5.

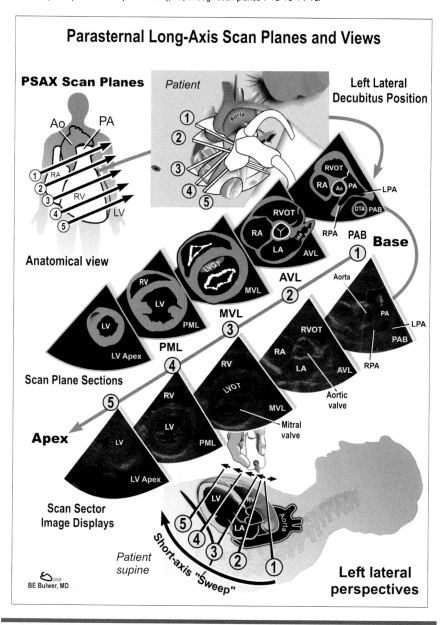

Parasternal Long-Axis Scan Planes and Views

PARASTENAL SHORT-AXIS (PSAX) VIEWS

The family of PSAX views provide important cross-sectional insights into cardiac chamber and valvular structure and function. At each level, the emphasis varies according to the region or structures of interest.

Patient and transducer positioning

For all PSAX views, the patient's position remains unchanged in the left lateral decubitus position. From the PLAX view, with the aortic valve (AV) in focus, rotate the transducer 90° clockwise to bring the short axis of the aortic valve into focus Figures 6.49–6.52 . The scan plane is oriented along a line drawn from the patient's right loin or hip region to the left shoulder.

Transducer maneuvers

The reference plane for the commencement of the PSAX views is the aortic valve level (PSAX-AVL) Figures 6.49, 6.50 . This is a preferred starting point, as the PSAX-AVL view is easily reproducible when maneuvering from the PLAX view. During diastolic closure, the characteristic Y-pattern of the aortic valve cups is seen Figures 6.53, 6.54 . To navigate the PSAX views, sweep or slide the transducer scan plane from the base of the heart superiorly toward the cardiac apex inferiorly. From the PLAX view, with the long axis of the aortic root and aortic valve in focus, clockwise rotation of the transducer plane 90° delivers the parasternal short-axis view at the aortic valve level (PSAX-AVL)—scan plane 2. This serves as a navigational reference plane for the PSAX views, from which subsequent PSAX views (1, 3, 4, and 5) are scanned. **1.** PSAX: Pulmonary Artery Bifurcation (PSAX-PAB); **2.** PSAX: Aortic valve level (PSAX-AVL); **3.** PSAX: Mitral valve level (PSAX-MVL); **4.** PSAX: Papillary Muscle Level (PSAX-PML); **5.** PSAX: Left Ventricular Apical Level (PSAX-Apical) Figure 6.50 . Sliding movements are recommended to minimize off-axis measurements of the left ventricular walls Figure 6.58 .

Transducer scan plane orientation and anatomy

The PSAX scan planes, when properly aligned, lie parallel to the plane of the cardiac base, and they are aligned perpendicular to the long-axis plane of the LV. The scan plane anatomy reflects the level of the short-axis scan plane Figure 6.50 .

M-Mode Examination

M-mode examination of the PSAX view is not routine, but it can be used to assess valve leaflet behavior, as well as linear dimensions of cardiac chambers and valves. M-mode of the RV outflow tract is used to assess diastolic collapse of the RVOT (on the PSAX-AVL view) in the setting of a pericardial effusion and suspected cardiac tamponade. See Figure 6.33 .

Color flow Doppler and spectral Doppler examination

Systematically examine all cardiac valves at each level. Focus on each valve individually, and examine valve structure and function—annulus, cusps, leaflets, commissures, mobility. Next, interrogate each valve using the sequence Figures 6.55–6.57 . See Figures 4.13, 4.21 . color flow Doppler → PW Doppler → CW Doppler. Apply the same approach when examining suspected or existing congenital or acquired heart disease, e.g., atrial and ventricular septal defects (VSD) or a patent ductus arteriosus (PDA). See Figures 6.34, 6.44 .

Coronary artery segments visualized on the PSAX view

Correlate ventricular wall motion abnormalities with their corresponding coronary artery supply. Corroborate such findings with complementary views Figures 6.23, 6.65 .

Findings: PSAX views

Assess cardiac structure and function as the examination proceeds. Use a systematic approach. Confirm normal and abnormal findings using subsequent views Tables 6.4, 6.5 .

PSAX VIEW: PATIENT POSITIONING, TRANSDUCER PLACEMENT, AND SCAN PLANE

Figure 6.51

Patient and transducer positioning: parasternal short-axis view (PSAX).

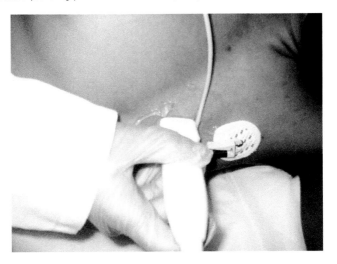

Figure 6.52

PSAX VIEW: aortic valve level.

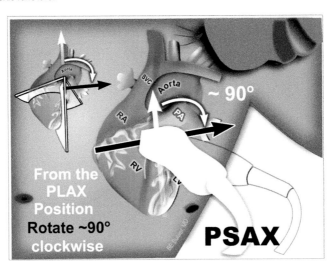

PSAX-AORTIC VALVE LEVEL (PSAX-AVL) VIEW

This view is for examination and assessment of the aortic valve (AV), pulmonary valve (PV), tricuspid valve (TV), right ventricular outflow tract (RVOT), main pulmonary artery (PA), left and right atria, and the interatrial septum (IAS).

Transducer scan plane orientation and anatomy

See Figures 6.51–6.53 . To optimize this view, ensure that the AV, PV, and TV are seen in one plane.

2D scan sector image display

Identify, optimize, and record the structures shown in Figures 6.53, 6.54 . Note the important anatomical relationships at the base of the heart. Note the diastolic closure Y-pattern ("inverted Mercedes-Benz" symbol) of the aortic cups and their relations. The right coronary cusp (rcc) lies between the septal leaflet of the tricuspid valve (TV) and the pulmonary valve (PV) leaflet; the left coronary cusp (lcc) is between the pulmonary valve and the left atrium (LA); the noncoronary cusp has its convexity attached perpendicular to the interatrial septum (IAS).

Measurements

- RVOT diameter measurement: most accurate on the PSAX-AVL view just proximal to the pulmonary valve Table 12.5
- Left atrial (LA) diameter (systole): on 2D guided M-mode, but PLAX and A4C linear measures, areas, and volumes are recommended Table 12.6

Valve Exam Protocol: 2D → Color Doppler → PW Doppler → CW Doppler

- **Aortic valve (AV):** Focus on the AV. Decrease depth (or zoom the AV). Examine valvular structures, namely the annulus, cusps, and commissures, for mobility, thickening, calcification, vegetations. Obtain 2D or M-mode linear dimensions if necessary Figures 6.53, 6.54 , and then interrogate by color Doppler to evaluate for possible aortic regurgitation (AR). The perpendicular alignment of the Doppler beam to the AV precludes spectral Doppler assessment.
- **Tricuspid valve (TV):** Apply color Doppler across the tricuspid valve, then PW Doppler to the leaflet tips for transvalvular RV inflow (optional), followed by CW Doppler to assess tricuspid regurgitation (TR) jet if present Figure 6.55 . Assess peak TR velocity (V_{max}) and derive pressure gradient using the Bernoulli equation ($p = 4v^2$) and corresponding PASP (as on the RV inflow view).
- **Pulmonary valve (PV):** Apply color flow Doppler to the RVOT and PV to assess for subpulmonary or pulmonary stenosis (PS), pulmonary regurgita-

tion (PR), or a patent ductus arteriosus (PDA). Apply PW Doppler and CW Doppler to PV or to other regions as applicable. For PR, measure diastolic velocities and derived pressures `Figures 4.5, 6.42, 6.48a`. For PS, measure peak and mean systolic velocities (V_{max} and V_{mean}) and derived peak and mean PA pressures (P_{max} and P_{mean}) `Figure 6.48b`.

- **Interatrial septum (IAS):** Focus on the IAS, and interrogate with color flow Doppler for suspected patent foramen ovale (PFO) or atrial septal defect (ASD).

Findings and Summaries

Assess cardiac structure and function. Confirm on complementary views `Table 6.4`.

PSAX VIEW—AORTIC VALVE LEVEL (AVL): SCAN PLANE AND SCAN SECTOR ANATOMY
Figure 6.53

Scan plane anatomy and scan sector displays of the PSAX-AVL view. Note the "Y" orientation of the AV valve cusps and their relationships to the tricuspid and pulmonary valves.

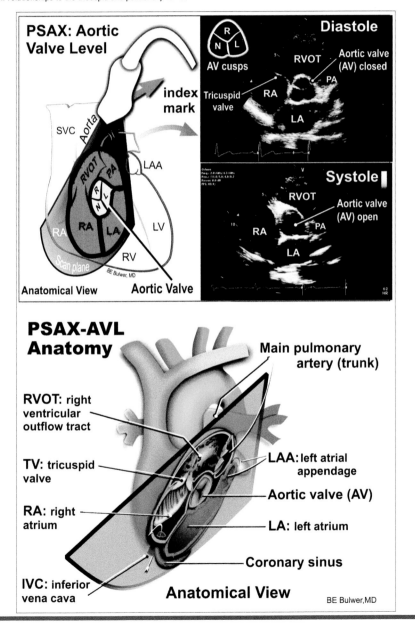

Figure 6.54

Scan sector frame showing structures visualized on the PSAX-AVL view.

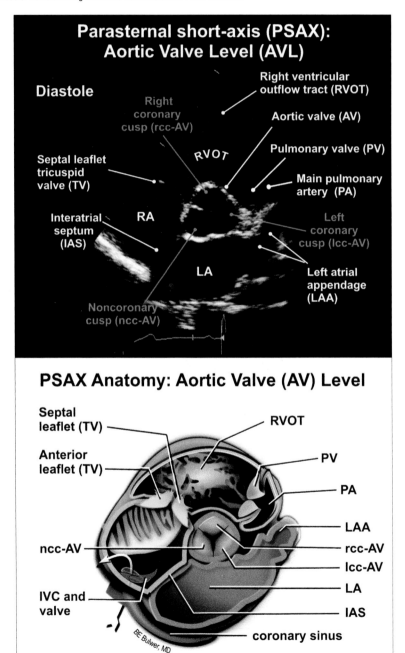

Parasternal short-axis (PSAX): Aortic Valve Level (AVL)

Diastole

Right ventricular outflow tract (RVOT)

Right coronary cusp (rcc-AV)

Aortic valve (AV)

Pulmonary valve (PV)

RVOT

Septal leaflet tricuspid valve (TV)

Main pulmonary artery (PA)

Interatrial septum (IAS)

RA

Left coronary cusp (lcc-AV)

LA

Left atrial appendage (LAA)

Noncoronary cusp (ncc-AV)

PSAX Anatomy: Aortic Valve (AV) Level

Septal leaflet (TV)

RVOT

Anterior leaflet (TV)

PV

PA

LAA

ncc-AV

rcc-AV

lcc-AV

LA

IVC and valve

IAS

coronary sinus

BE Bulwer, MD

PSAX VIEW—AVL: DOPPLER EXAM—TRICUSPID VALVE
Figure 6.55

Parasternal short-axis (PSAX): aortic valve level. *Top panel.* Color flow Doppler to the tricuspid valve (TV). *Middle panel.* PW Doppler time velocity profile of the TV inflow, showing early (E) and late (A) diastolic flow velocities. *Bottom panel.* Color flow-guided CW Doppler to assess TR velocities.

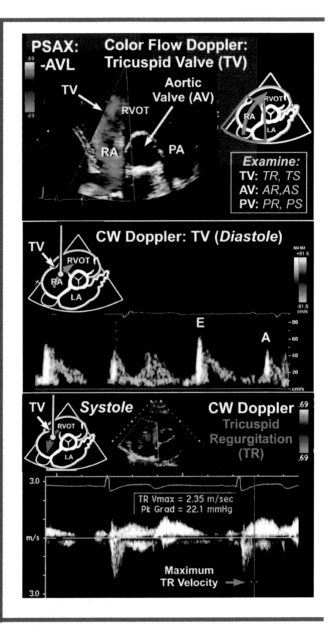

PSAX VIEW—PULMONARY ARTERY BIFURCATION (PAB): SCAN SECTOR ANATOMY

Figure 6.56

PSAX-PAB scan sector image display and cross-sectional anatomy.

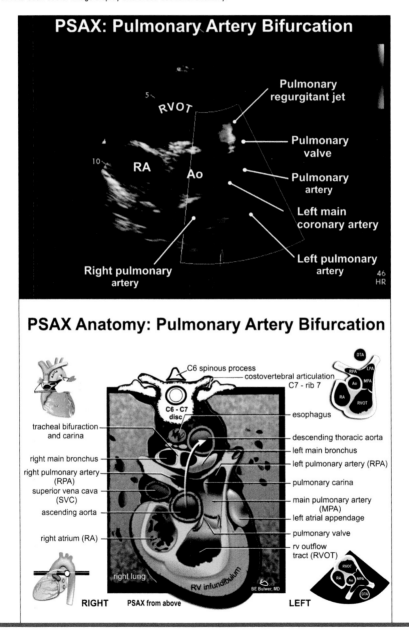

PSAX—PULMONARY ARTERY BIFURCATION (PSAX-PAB)

This view is useful for evaluating the main pulmonary artery (PA), the pulmonary valve (PV), the right and left pulmonary arteries, origins of the left main and right coronary arteries, and patent ductus arteriosus (PDA) Figures 6.56, 6.57 .

Transducer maneuvers, scan plane, and anatomy

From the PSAX-AVL view, slightly angulate the transducer scan plane superiorly above the level of the aortic valve cusps Figures 6.49, 6.50, 6.56 . Adjust to optimize visualization of the PA bifurcation and associated structures. Slight degrees of clockwise rotations should bring the right (RCA) and left main (LCA) coronary arteries into view as they exit the aorta and enter the right and left atrioventricular grooves. The RCA originates at ~11 o'clock position, and the LCA originates at ~4 o'clock position, of the aortic root Figure 6.56 .

2D scan sector image display

Identify, optimize, and record the structures shown in Figure 6.56 .

Color flow and spectral (PW, CW) Doppler exam

Sequentially examine the PV or other regions of interest using a systematic approach: color flow Doppler → PW Doppler → CW Doppler Figure 6.57 .

Normal findings: PSAX: PB

Assess cardiac structure and function. Confirm normal and abnormal findings on complementary views Table 6.4 .

PSAX VIEW—PAB: DOPPLER EXAM—PULMONARY VALVE
Figure 6.57

Upper panel. Systolic still frame showing color flow Doppler examination of the main pulmonary artery and its bifurcation on the PSAX-PAB view. Note the blue color flow velocities directed away from the transducer. *Lower panel.* Color-guided PW and CW Doppler interrogation of the pulmonary valve. Note systolic spectral Doppler velocities below the baseline. Mild degrees of pulmonary regurgitation (PR) are present in most normal individuals. On the 2D guide and sketch, note the red diastolic PR jet directed toward the transducer and the corresponding spectral Doppler velocities displayed above the baseline.

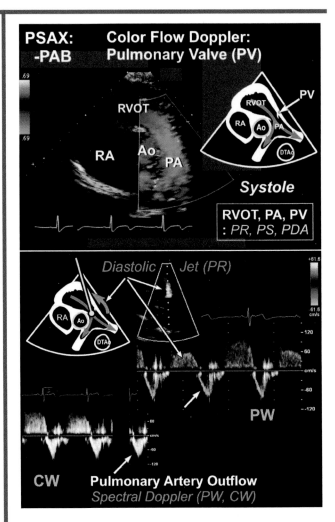

PSAX VIEW—AVL AND PAB: NORMAL AND ABNORMAL FINDINGS

Table 6.4 PARASTENAL SHORT-AXIS (PSAX) VIEWS—AORTIC VALVE AND PULMONARY ARTERY BIFURCATION LEVELS: THE EXAMINATION SURVEY

Sequential survey	Abnormalities visualized in the parasternal short-axis (PSAX) view—aortic valve level (AVL)/pulmonary artery bifurcation (PAB)	
	Structural: on 2D, 3D, or M-mode	Functional and hemodynamic (on Doppler, including color Doppler)
Aortic valve (AV)	Corroborate findings with the PLAX view; see Table 6.1 ; Figs. 6.27–6.29 • Aortic annuli or leaflet pathology: aortic stenosis (AS), bicuspid, unicuspid, or quadricuspid aortic valves • Calcification: leaflet, annulus, commissures • Leaflet mobility • Aortic root dilatation • Sinus of Valsalva aneurysm • Aortic dissection-flap • Vegetations: infective endocarditis • Mass/tumor, e.g., papillary fibroelastoma • Prosthetic aortic valve • Coronary arteries—left main AORTIC VALVE LEVEL • Coronary arteries: dilatation, calcification, or aneurysm	Corroborate findings with the PLAX view; see Table 6.1 ; Figs. 6.27–6.29 Color flow Doppler • AR jet in diastole (jet ratio) • Systolic turbulence in AS Ventricular septal defects (VSD): Short-axis orientation • Gerbode type: LV to RA—8 or 9 o'clock position • Membranous—10 o'clock position • Outlet-infracristal—12 o'clock position • Outlet-supracristal—2 o'clock position AORTIC REGURGITATION (AR) • Assess etiology • Estimate severity: mild, moderate, severe Fig. 6.28 AORTIC STENOSIS (AS) • Assess etiology • Estimate severity: mild, moderate, severe Figs. 4.15, 6.29, 10.2
Right atrium (RA)	• Corroborate findings with the RV inflow view; see Table 6.2 ; Fig. 6.44 • RA enlargement (dilatation) • R atrial masses—most commonly thrombi • Chiari network (embryonic remnant of the sinus venosum— nonpathologic) • Cardiac hardware, e.g., pacemaker/defibrillator wire— traverses tricuspid valve	Corroborate findings with the RV inflow view; see Table 6.2 • Tricuspid regurgitation (TR) jet on color flow Doppler Fig. 6.43a • Elevated right atrial pressures (RAP) Figs. 4.5, 6.42 ; Table 8.1 • VSD—Gerbode type defect (LV to RA) on color flow and spectral Doppler

(continues)

Table 6.4 PARASTENAL SHORT-AXIS (PSAX) VIEWS—AORTIC VALVE AND PULMONARY ARTERY BIFURCATION LEVELS: THE EXAMINATION SURVEY *(continued)*

Sequential survey	Abnormalities visualized in the parasternal short-axis (PSAX) view—aortic valve level (AVL)/pulmonary artery bifurcation (PAB)	
	Structural: on 2D, 3D, or M-mode	Functional and hemodynamic (on Doppler, including color Doppler)
Right ventricular outflow tract (RVOT) and **Pulmonary artery (PA)**	Corroborate findings with the PLAX, RV inflow and outflow views; see Tables 6.1, 6.2, 6.3 RVOT CAVITY • Dilatation, e.g., in pressure or volume overload states • Wall thickness PA TRUNK • Dilatation, e.g., in pressure or volume overload states • PA banding—residual from previous intervention in congenital heart disease MEASUREMENTS: RVOT and PA Table 12.5 • RVOT diameters • PA diameter	Corroborate findings with the PLAX, RV inflow and outflow views; see Tables 6.1, 6.2, 6.3 RVOT WALL • Diastolic collapse with pericardial effusion/tamponade— confirm on M-mode Patent ductus arteriosus (PDA): assess on color flow and spectral Doppler See also Figs. 6.31–6.33, 6.48a, 6.48b
Pulmonary valve (PV)	• Thickened immobile leaflets in carcinoid syndrome • Pulmonary artery bifurcation Fig. 6.58 : thromboemboli, stenosis, dilatation	PULMONARY REGURGITATION (PR) • Assess etiology • Estimate severity: mild, moderate, severe Fig. 6.48a PULMONARY STENOSIS (PS) • Assess etiology • Estimate severity: mild, moderate, severe Fig. 6.48b
Right (RPA) and left (LPA) pulmonary artery	• Thickened in chronic overload states, e.g., chronic pulmonary hypertension • Saddle embolus (pulmonary embolism)	• Patent ductus arteriosus (PDA)—aorta-to-left pulmonary artery (LPA) flow: assess on color flow and spectral Doppler
Left atrium (LA)	Corroborate findings with the PLAX and A4C views; see Tables 6.1, 7.2 • LA enlargement (dilatation) • Left atrial tumor—most commonly a myxoma • Left atrial appendage ± clot	Corroborate findings with the PLAX and A4C views; see Tables 6.1, 7.2 • Atrial fibrillation (loss of atrial contraction) • Spontaneous echocontrast "smoke" (best seen on TEE) • ASD on color flow Doppler
Interatrial septum	• Patent foramen ovale (PFO) • Atrial septal defect (ASD) Fig. 6.44	• Color flow Doppler assessment • Subcostal view best for assessment of PFO/ASD Fig. 8.9a • Agitated saline "bubble" study on A4C view

PSAX VIEW: RECOMMENDED SCANNING TECHNIQUE
Figure 6.58

Two-dimensional echocardiography, being operator dependent, is not a true tomographic technique compared to cardiac computerized tomography (CT) and cardiac MRI. It is therefore prone to off-axis imaging during the examination. When obtaining short-axis ventricular dimensions, sliding *(lower-panel)* rather than angulation techniques *(upper panel)* result in orthogonal cross-sectional scans. Optimally acquired short-axis views of the LV should appear round, rather than oval, when slices are oriented orthogonal to the LV long axis.

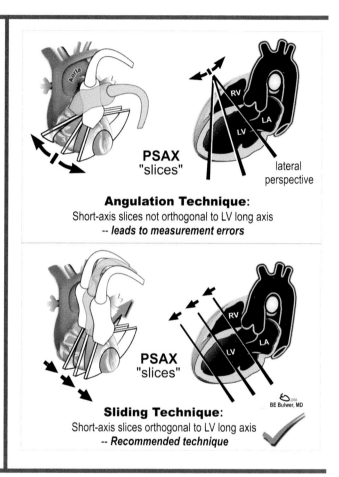

PSAX "slices"

lateral perspective

Angulation Technique:
Short-axis slices not orthogonal to LV long axis
-- leads to measurement errors

PSAX "slices"

BE Bulwer, MD

Sliding Technique:
Short-axis slices orthogonal to LV long axis
-- Recommended technique

PSAX VIEW—MITRAL VALVE LEVEL (PSAX-MVL)

The primary focus is the mitral valve (MV), the surrounding basal walls of the left ventricle (LV) including the basal interventricular septum (IVS), and the LV outflow tract (LVOT). The right ventricle (RV), its outflow tract (RVOT), and the tricuspid valve (TV) are usually imaged in this view.

Transducer maneuvers and scan plane orientation

From the PSAX-AVL view, slightly slide or angulate the transducer toward the LV apex until the primary structures of interest are visualized [Figures 6.59, 6.60]. Ensure scan plane is oriented perpendicular to the LV long axis, with the LV walls appearing circular rather than oval. Note the normal crescent-shaped RV-RVOT.

2D scan sector image display

Identify, optimize, and record the structures shown in [Figures 6.59, 6.60].

- **Mitral valve:** Note the characteristic "fish mouth" appearance of the mitral valve orifice. Examine MV leaflets. Identify the anterior and posterior mitral leaflet and mitral scallops (Carpentier nomenclature) [Figures 6.24, 6.61]. This has implications for surgical intervention, especially when describing leaflet and scallop involvement in mitral regurgitation (MR) [Figure 6.25]. However, transesophageal echocardiography (TEE) is the standard for optimal assessment of the mitral valve. The LVOT describes the region at the level of, and superior to, the MV level, where its boundaries are the basal interventricular septum, the anterior leaflet of the mitral valve. Planimetry of the mitral valve orifice area—measured at the tips of the mitral leaflets—is performed in mitral stenosis [Figure 6.26].
- **Left ventricle (LV):** Optional measures—basal LV size, function, and wall thicknesses [Figures 6.18–6.23].
- **Right ventricle (RV):** Assess RV cavity size and function [Figures 6.31, 6.32]. The cross-sectional diameter of the RV is normally ~ 2/3 that of the LV at this point.

M-mode exam

M-mode of the PSAX views of mitral valve is an option to the standard using the PLAX view. It can confirm diastolic fluttering of the anterior mitral leaflet in aortic regurgitation (AR) [Figure 6.28].

Color flow Doppler exam

Its use is limited, but it can show accelerated diastolic flow (mosaic pattern) at the MV orifice in mitral stenosis (MS) [Figure 6.26], or the vena contracta of the systolic jet of mitral regurgitation (MR) [Figure 6.25], or diastolic fluttering of the anterior mitral leaflet in AR because of the presence of a posteriorly directed jet.

Spectral Doppler exam

The perpendicular Doppler angle alignment precludes spectral Doppler assessment.

Coronary artery segments visualized on the PLAX view

Identify basal LV segments, and correlate abnormalities of basal ventricular wall motion and thickening with their corresponding coronary artery supply [Figures 6.23, 6.65].

Findings and Summaries

Assess cardiac structure and function. Confirm findings on complementary views [Table 6.5].

PSAX VIEW—MITRAL VALVE LEVEL (MVL): SCAN PLANE AND SCAN SECTOR ANATOMY

Figure 6.59

Parasternal short-axis view: mitral valve level (PSAX-MVL) scan plane *(left)* and scan sector frames during diastole and systole (*right* panels).

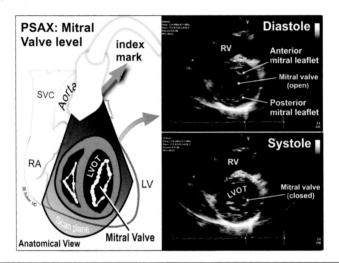

Figure 6.60

PSAX-MVL scan sector image display and cross-sectional anatomy.

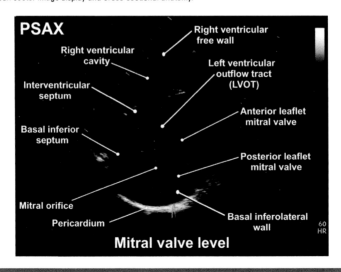

PSAX VIEW—SURGICAL CONSIDERATIONS: MITRAL VALVE SCALLOPS
Figure 6.61

Anatomical perspectives of mitral valve leaflets and scallops *(upper panel)* and the corresponding surgical *views (lower panel)*. Although transesophageal echocardiography—both 2D and 3D—plays an essential role in the evaluation of mitral valve leaflet and scallops in the perioperative setting, transthoracic echocardiography still plays a foundational role. The classification shown is the Carpentier classification of the mitral valve scallops. The Duran classification is preferred by some surgeons.

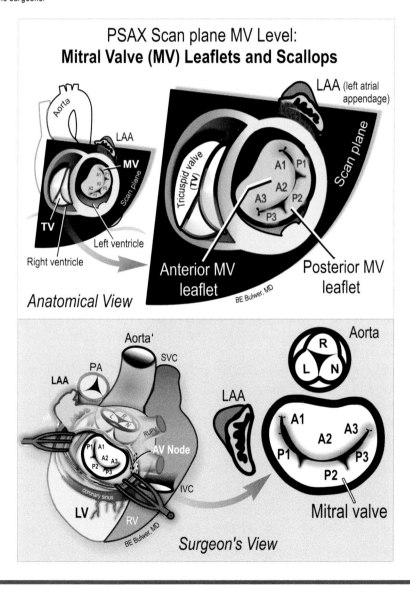

PSAX VIEW—PAPILLARY MUSCLE LEVEL (PSAX-PML)

The region of interest is the mid-left ventricular (LV) walls, with a pair of papillary muscles, the mid-interventricular septum (IVS), and the right ventricle (RV).

Transducer maneuvers and scan plane orientation

From the PSAX-MVL view, slightly slide or angulate the transducer toward the LV apex until the primary structures of interest are visualized Figures 6.62, 6.63 . Ensure perpendicular alignment, with the LV short axis appearing circular, not oval.

2D scan sector image display

Identify, optimize, and record the structures shown in Figures 6.63–6.65 .

- **Left ventricle (LV):** Identify LV segments. Assess LV size, wall thicknesses, and regional LV function. Correlate with other LV segments.
- **Papillary muscles:** Identify anterolateral and posterolateral papillary muscles (at approximately the 4 o'clock and 8 o'clock positions) and their corresponding inferolateral and inferior LV segments, respectively Figures 6.63–6.65 .
- **Right ventricle (RV):** Assess RV cavity size and function.

M-mode exam

M-mode of the PSAX views just beyond the tips of the mitral leaflets is an alternative to the standard of using the PLAX view.

Color flow Doppler exam

Its use is limited, but interrogate the interventricular septum for possible ventricular septal defect (VSD) Figure 6.34 .

Spectral Doppler exam

The perpendicular Doppler angle alignment precludes spectral Doppler assessment, unless there is a muscular VSD or lesion oriented appropriately.

Coronary artery segments visualized on the PSAX view

Identify mid-LV segments, and correlate abnormalities of mid-ventricular wall motion and thickening with their corresponding coronary artery supply Figures 6.43, 6.65 .

Findings and Summaries

Assess cardiac structure and function. Confirm findings on complementary views Table 6.5 .

PSAX VIEW—APICAL LEVEL (PSAX-APICAL)

Transducer maneuvers and scan plane orientation

From the PSAX-PML view, slightly slide or angulate the transducer to visualize LV apex and the apical cap (with no LV lumen).

Findings and Summaries: 2D Scan Sector Image Display, Doppler Examination, and Coronary Artery Segments

Follow the same protocol and principles as for assessment of the PSAX-PML view.

PSAX VIEW—PAPILLARY MUSCLE LEVEL (MVL): SCAN PLANE AND SCAN SECTOR ANATOMY

Figure 6.62

Parasternal short axis (PSAX) view: mid-ventricle/papillary muscle level.

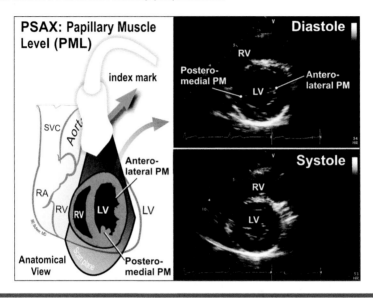

Figure 6.63

Scan sector frames and cross-sectional anatomy at the papillary muscle (PSAX-PML) and apical (PSAX-Apical) levels.

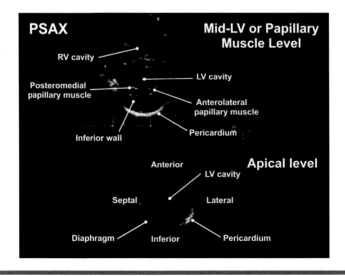

PSAX VIEW: 3D PERSPECTIVES
Figure 6.64

Parasternal acquisition of three-dimensional (3D) pyramidal full-volume data set cropped to display the parasternal short-axis (PSAX) plane in real time. Short-axis cropped planes are useful for assessing the atrioventricular valves and ventricular structure and function (see Figures 2.6, 2.7, 6.11, 7.12).

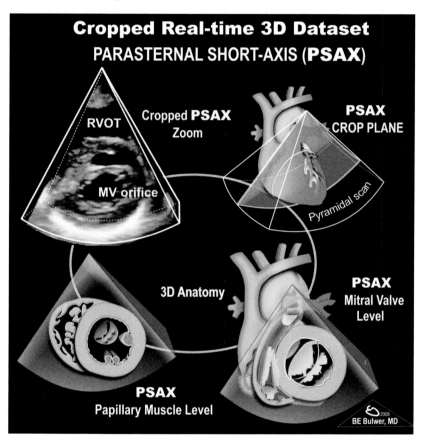

PSAX VIEWS AND CORONARY ARTERY TERRITORIES
Figure 6.65

The parasternal short-axis (PSAX) view and corresponding coronary artery territories and LV segments. Compare with Figures 2.9, 6.10, 6.23, 7.13.

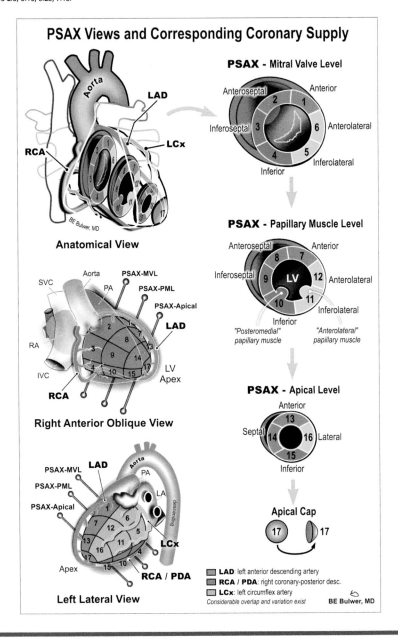

PSAX VIEW—MITRAL VALVE AND LEFT VENTRICULAR LEVELS: NORMAL AND ABNORMAL FINDINGS

Table 6.4 . Possible Findings and Assessments in the PSAX Windows in Adults: Mitral Valve and Ventricular Levels.

Table 6.5 PARASTERNAL SHORT-AXIS VIEW—MITRAL VALVE (PSAX-MVL) AND LEFT VENTRICULAR LEVELS: THE EXAMINATION SURVEY

Sequential survey	Abnormalities visualized in the parasternal short-axis (PSAX) view: mitral valve and ventricular levels	
	Structural: on 2D, 3D, or M-mode	Functional and hemodynamic
Mitral valve (MV) level	Corroborate findings with the PLAX and A4C views; see Tables 6.1, 7.2 MV STRUCTURE: leaflet scallops Figs. 6.24, 6.61 MV LEAFLET MOBILITY MITRAL VALVE SCORING CRITERIA IN MITRAL STENOSIS (MS) • Leaflet mobility • Subvalvular thickening • Valve leaflet thickening • Calcification MV PROLAPSE: (one or both leaflets) MV PLANIMETRY IN MS for MV AREA (MVA) Fig. 6.26 • Confirm with Doppler measures • Normal MVA: 4–6 cm^2 LVOT (left ventricular outflow tract) • Assymetric septal hypertrophy • Systolic anterior motion of the mitral valve (SAM) LV WALL STRUCTURE: BASAL • LV walls visualized and assessed: basal LV walls Figs. 6.21, 6.22, 6.60, 6.61, 6.65	Corroborate findings with the PLAX and A4C views; see Tables 6.1, 7.2 MV DYNAMICS • Systolic anterior motion (SAM) of the mitral valve ± dynamic LVOT obstruction (confirm on M-mode) • Diastolic fluttering of anterior mitral leaflet (AML) ± premature MV closure in aortic regurgitation (AR) MITRAL REGURGITATION (MR) • Assess etiology • Estimate severity: mild, moderate, severe Fig. 6.25 MITRAL STENOSIS (MS) • Assess etiology • Estimate severity: mild, moderate, severe Fig. 6.26 LV WALL MOTION and WALL THICKENING: BASAL LV • Wall motion score (WMS) and WMS index Figs. 6.21, 6.22 • Correlate with corresponding coronary artery blood supply Figs. 6.23, 6.60, 6.61, 6.65
Left ventricular (LV) level	Corroborate findings with the PLAX and A4C views; see Tables 6.1, 7.2 LV CAVITY Table 12.1 • Cavity size: normal, increased, decreased • LV enlargement (dilatation)	Corroborate findings with the PLAX and A4C views; see Tables 6.1, 7.2 LV SYSTOLIC FUNCTION ASSESSMENT • Summary measures Figs. 6.18–6.23

(continues)

Table 6.5 PARASTERNAL SHORT-AXIS VIEW—MITRAL VALVE (PSAX-MVL) AND LEFT VENTRICULAR LEVELS: THE EXAMINATION SURVEY *(continued)*

Sequential survey	Abnormalities visualized in the parasternal short-axis (PSAX) view: mitral valve and ventricular levels	
	Structural: on 2D, 3D, or M-mode	Functional and hemodynamic
	LV WALL STRUCTURE: BASAL, MID-LV, and APICAL LEVELS • LV walls visualized and assessed: Figs. 6.21, 6.22, 6.60, 6.63, 6.65 • LV hypertrophy including hypertrophic cardiomyopathy (HCM)Interventricular septum— VSD: inlet, muscular (trabecular) Fig. 6.34 PAPILLARY MUSCLE LEVEL • Papillary muscles: number, disposition, displacement, rupture • Anterolateral papillary muscle (~4 o'clock position); postero-medial papillary muscle (~8 o'clock position) APICAL LEVEL Figs. 6.63, 6.65 • Aneurysm • Masses: thrombus, tumor • Apical hypertrophic cardio-myopathy • LV noncompaction	LV CAVITY Table 12.2 • Systolic dysfunction /RWMA/ impaired contractility, e.g., post MI; cardiomyopathies; decom-pensated valvular heart disease LV WALL MOTION and WALL THICKENING: BASAL, MID-LV, and APICAL LEVELS • Wall motion score (WMS) and WMS index Figs. 6.21, 6.22 • Correlate with corresponding coronary artery blood supply Figs. 6.23, 6.60, 6.63, 6.65 LV WALL (SEPTUM) • LV dyssynchrony (on M-mode) • Paradoxical movement and "D-shaped septum," e.g., in right ventricular pressure and volume overload states—pulmonary hy-pertension; L-to-R shunts, e.g., secundum ASD Figs. 6.31, 6.32 • Constrictive pericarditis—"septal bounce" Fig. 6.33
Right ventricle (RV)	Corroborate findings with the PLAX view; see Table 6.1 RV/RVOT CAVITY • Dilatation, e.g., in pressure or volume overload states, e.g., right heart failure; primary and secondary pulmonary hypertension; secundum ASD Figs. 6.31, 6.32 • Pacemaker or defibrillator wire RV/RVOT WALL • Thickened in chronic overload states, e.g., chronic pulmonary hypertension • Masses, thrombus RV DIMENSIONS, AREAS, VOLUMES: Figs. 6.31, 6.32 ; Tables 12.4, 12.5	Corroborate findings with the PLAX view; see Table 6.1 RV/RVOT CAVITY • Systolic dysfunction/impaired contractility, e.g., in RV pressure and volume overload states RV/RVOT WALL • Diastolic collapse with pericar-dial effusion/tamponade—confirm on M-mode Fig. 6.33 RV FUNCTION MEASURES Fig. 6.32 ; Table 12.4
Pericardium	• Pericardial effusion • Pericardial thickening: corroborate findings with the PLAX view; see Table 6.1 ; Fig. 6.33	• ± tamponade physiology • ± constrictive physiology • Findings consistent with tampon-ade—including RV diastolic collapse Fig. 6.33

CHAPTER 7

Apical Windows, Views, and Scan Planes

Figure 7.1

A family of apical scan planes as viewed from both the anatomical position and with the patient in the left lateral decubitus position.

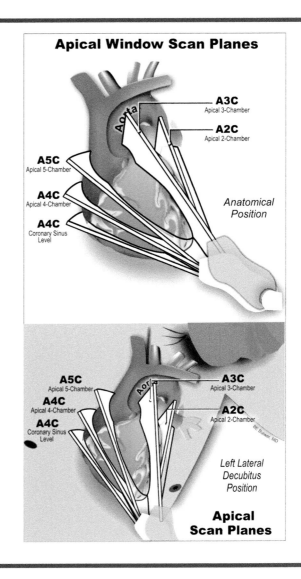

Apical Window Scan Planes

- **A3C** Apical 3-Chamber
- **A2C** Apical 2-Chamber
- **A5C** Apical 5-Chamber
- **A4C** Apical 4-Chamber
- **A4C** Coronary Sinus Level

Aorta

Anatomical Position

- **A5C** Apical 5-Chamber
- **A4C** Apical 4-Chamber
- **A4C** Coronary Sinus Level
- **A3C** Apical 3-Chamber
- **A2C** Apical 2-Chamber

Aorta

Left Lateral Decubitus Position

Apical Scan Planes

APICAL WINDOWS AND VIEWS

The apical windows, along with the parasternal views, are the most commonly used in the transthoracic examination. The apical views are obtained by scanning from the true cardiac apex toward the base Figure 7.1 . The primary apical views are:

- Apical four-chamber (A4C) view Figures 7.1–7.26
- Apical five-chamber (A5C) view Figures 7.1, 7.4, 7.27–7.31
- Apical two-chamber (A2C) view Figures 7.1, 7.32–7.37
- Apical three-chamber (A3C) or long-axis (ALAX) view Figures 7.1, 7.38–7.43

The apical views, particularly the A4C view, are indispensable for assessing global and regional ventricular function.

Patient and transducer positioning

As for the PSAX views, the left lateral decubitus position is preferred, as gravity displaces the cardiac apex closer to the chest wall Figures 6.51, 6.52 . Using a cutout mattress may further facilitate transducer maneuvers.

Transducer maneuvers

Although the site of maximal apical impulse can assist in locating the true anatomic LV apex, it often fails to correspond, and LV foreshortening Figure 7.7 results.

Identifying the true LV apex on echocardiography

On the 2D examination, the true LV apex can be identified by:

- Stepwise location and identification of the apical cap on the PSAX views, followed by steep orthogonal angulation up toward the base.
- The wall of the true LV apex is thinner than the remainder of the LV walls. From the true LV apex, the desired views: A4C→A5C→A2C→A3C are obtained by both angulation and anticlockwise rotation of the transducer along the planes as shown Figures 7.1–7.4 .
- Relative immobility: the true cardiac apex appears relatively stationary compared to the rest of the ventricular walls.
- Accurate 3D-guided identification of the true LV apex. This, and subsequent calculation of linear and volumetric measures, e.g., LV mass and volumes, are among the advantages of 3D echocardiography Figures 6.18, 6.20 .

2D scan sector image display

There are two widely used display options for the A4C (and A5C) views Figures 7.4–7.12 . In adult echocardiography, the most popular is the "apex up" projection with the apex shown at the top of the scan sector display. In pediatric echocardiography, the "inverted" apex display is mostly used, with the apex displayed at the bottom of the scan sector in the apical and subcostal (subxiphoid) views (see Figures 7.5, 7.6, 7.10, 8.6). This facilitates the display and interpretation of structures in their correct anatomic orientation, which is an issue of special importance in pediatric cardiology and congenital heart disease. The apex up display has the advantage of being more consistent with the display formats used in computerized topography (CT), magnetic resonance imaging (MRI), and general radiology, where tomographic structures are displayed as viewed from below and toward the head Figures 7.4, 7.5 .

APICAL VIEWS: PATIENT POSITIONING AND TRANSDUCER PLACEMENT

Figure 7.2

Patient and transducer positioning: patient in the left lateral decubitus position with transducer placed at the apical window.

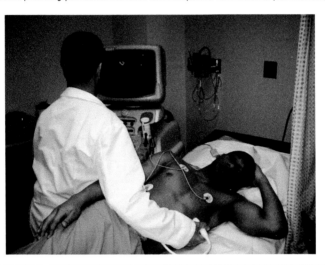

Figure 7.3

Zoomed view of the apical window and transducer orientation for obtaining A4C view. Note the direction of the transducer index mark (insert, black arrow). Compare with Figures 7.4–7.6.

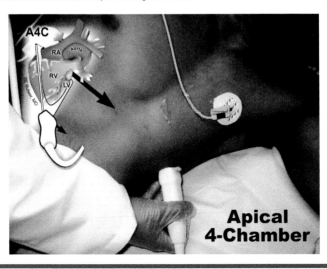

APICAL 4-CHAMBER AND 5-CHAMBER SCAN PLANES, ANATOMY, AND SCAN SECTOR DISPLAY
Figure 7.4

Family of apical four-chamber scan planes. *Upper left.* Sweeping from inferiorly to superiorly, the transducer scan plane moves from the level of the coronary sinus to the four-chamber plane (A4C), and to the five-chamber (A5C) plane. Note the direction of the index mark (red arrow). *Bottom.* Left lateral supine view of the A4C and A5C scan planes showing the primary structures that these planes transect. *Upper right.* The corresponding scan sector displays of the A4C and A5C views. Using this widely used projection format, the left ventricle (LV) is displayed on the same side as the transducer index mark (red arrows). Compare with the projections in Figures 7.5, 7.6.

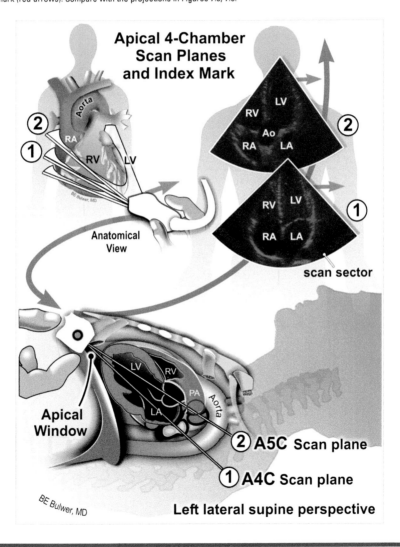

A4C: ANATOMICAL ORIENTATION
Figure 7.5

Anatomical projections of the apical four-chamber (A4C) scan plane (left and center). The widely used projection of the A4C view, as shown in Figures 2.6, 7.4, and 7.6, corresponds to the upper anatomical segment shown on the right. Compare with the projections shown in Figure 7.6. On 2D or cross-sectional echocardiography, this is not terribly important per se, as only a thin slice or cross section is displayed. However, it becomes important in 3D echocardiography, where out-of-plane anatomy is displayed. The heart is grossly asymmetric, and structures above the A4C scan plane are clearly different from those below.

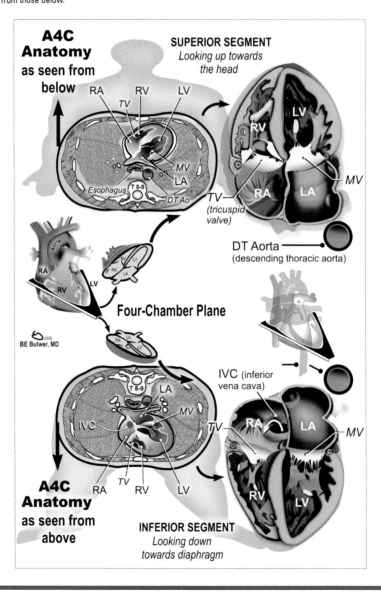

A4C VIEWS AND PROJECTIONS
Figure 7.6

A4C projections and image display options. The apex up view is most popular in adult echocardiography. The apex down projection is widely used in pediatric cardiology to define cardiac situs (site or location) in congenital heart disease. For apex up projections, there is an alternative "Mayo Clinic" presentation, where the left and right sides of the display are switched. Some may find this confusing, but a clear understanding of three-dimensional cardiac anatomy should relegate this to a mere matter of preference.

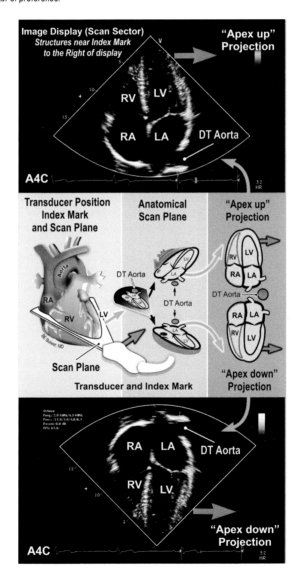

A4C: AVOIDANCE OF LV FORESHORTENING
Figure 7.7

Left ventricular foreshortening. Foreshortening *(shown right)* occurs when the imaging plane does not transect the true left ventricular apex *(left)*. It is a common source of error in left ventricular quantification in two-dimensional echocardiography. The true anatomical LV apical wall is thinner than the remainder of the LV wall.

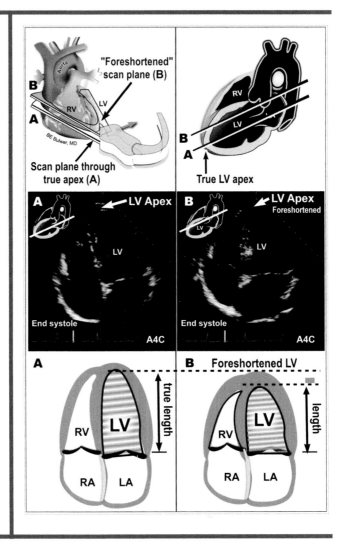

APICAL FOUR-CHAMBER (A4C) VIEW

The A4C view is used to assess LV apex, all four cardiac chambers (LA, LV, RA, and RV), and the atrioventricular valves (MV and TV). It is one of the most important standard planes, and it is central to the assessment of LV systolic and diastolic function.

Patient and transducer positioning

With patient lying in the left lateral position, or steeper if necessary, palpate the cardiac impulse and apply transducer (with coupling gel). Orient the transducer as shown Figures 7.2–7.4 .

Transducer maneuvers

With the patient in the left lateral decubitus position and the transducer positioned at the apical impulse and directed toward the right shoulder, and index mark at ~ 3 o'clock position, maneuver the scan plane until the primary structures shown in Figures 7.8 and 7.9 appear. Optimally align image:

- The LV apex should be at the apex of the scan sector with the LV long axis directed parallel to the transducer beam. This is important, as several key Doppler parameters are measured using the A4C view Figures 7.13, 7.26 ; Table 7.1 .
- Avoid LV foreshortening Figure 7.7 . LV quantification, e.g., areas, volumes, and mass, depend on accurate identification of the LV apex Figures 6.19–6.21 .
- Ensure that cardiac chambers are displayed at the recommended 4C plane, so that cardiac chambers are displayed with their maximal diameters. If the coronary sinus appears in the A4C display, the scan plane is too low (directed too inferiorly). If the aortic root is seen, the scan plane is too high.

2D scan sector image display

Scan at depths of 20–24 cm and visualize cardiac and extracardiac structures. Decrease depth to 15–16 cm for closer views of cardiac structures or other regions of interest. Identify, optimize, and record structures shown in Figures 7.8–7.11 .

   Assess and measure LV, LA, RV, and RA chamber size and function, including Simpson's rule Figures 6.18–6.23, 6.30, 6.31, 6.44 ; Tables 12.1–12.6 .

Doppler examination

- **Pulmonary vein (Pv) Inflow**→Color Doppler→PW Doppler Figures 7.17–7.18 ; Table 7.1 .
- **Mitral valve (MV)**→Transmitral LV Inflow: Color Doppler→PW Doppler→CW Doppler→color M-mode (flow propagation velocity) Figures 7.14–7.16, 7.19–7.20 ; Table 7.1 .

- **Mitral annulus (septal and lateral)**→Tissue Doppler Imaging of mitral annular (longitudinal) velocities `Figures 7.18–7.22`; `Table 7.1`.
- **Tricuspid valve (TV)**→Color Doppler→PW Doppler→CW Doppler `Figure 7.26`.

Coronary artery segments visualized on the PLAX view

Correlate abnormalities of ventricular wall motion and thickening with their corresponding coronary artery supply `Figures 2.9, 6.10, 6.23, 6.65, 7.13, 7.36, 7.42`.

Findings and Summaries

Assess cardiac structure and function. Confirm findings on complementary views `Table 7.2`.

A4C: SCAN SECTOR ANATOMY
Figure 7.8

Apical four-chamber (A4C) views: scan plane and scan sector displays.

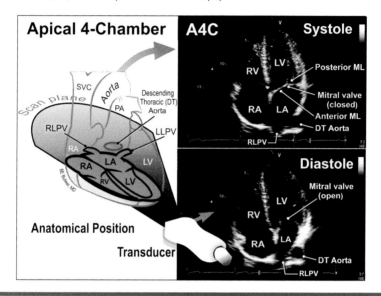

Figure 7.9

Scan sector systolic frame showing the cross-sectional anatomy of the apical four-chamber (A4C) view.

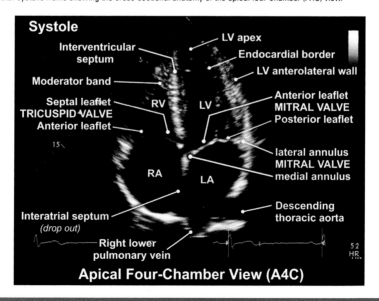

A4C: VENTRICULAR MORPHOLOGIC CRITERIA
Figure 7.10

The internal cardiac crux is where the internal septae and atrioventricular valves meet. Note the more apical insertion of the septal leaflet of the tricuspid valve (insert).

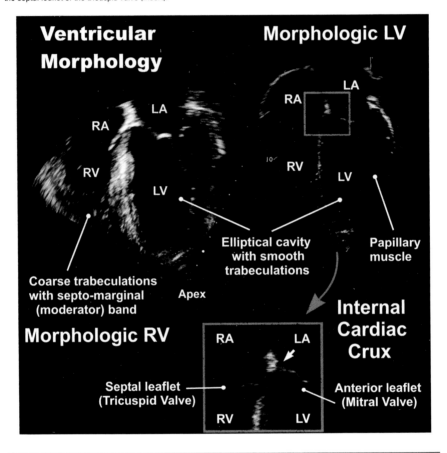

Figure 7.11

Defining morphological left and right ventricles on two-dimensional (2D) echocardiography. The confluence of the inter-ventricular and interatrial septa and the septal insertions of the tricuspid and mitral valve leaflets constitute the internal cardiac crux (cross). The normal cross-like configuration on 2D echocardiography is not symmetrical. The septal leaflet of the tricuspid valve is inserted more apically, i.e., toward the cardiac apex. This relationship becomes important in evaluating certain congenital heart lesions, e.g., atrioventricular canal defects. Another distinguishing echocardiographic feature of the morphological right ventricle is its coarser trabeculated endocardial surface (including the moderator band), the presence of a tricuspid valve, and the absence of two distinct papillary muscles. These characteristics are important in segmental sequential analysis of congenital heart disease (see Table 8.2).

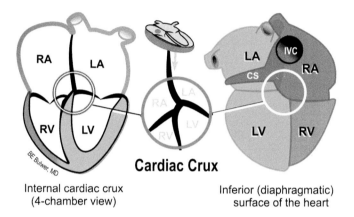

Cardiac Crux

Internal cardiac crux
(4-chamber view)

Inferior (diaphragmatic)
surface of the heart

Atrioventricular Canal (AVC) Defects

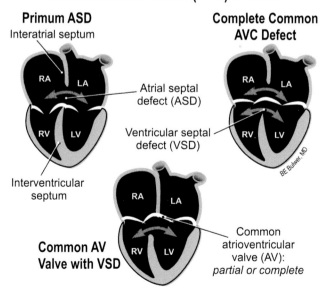

Primum ASD
Interatrial septum

Complete Common
AVC Defect

Atrial septal
defect (ASD)

Ventricular septal
defect (VSD)

Interventricular
septum

Common AV
Valve with VSD

Common
atrioventricular
valve (AV):
partial or complete

A4C: 3D PERSPECTIVES
Figure 7.12

Apical acquisition of three-dimensional (3D) pyramidal full-volume data set cropped to display the apical four-chamber (A4C) plane in real time (see Figures 2.6, 2.7, 6.11, 6.64).

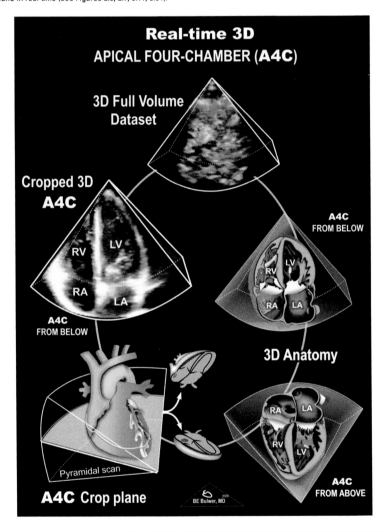

A4C: VIEW AND CORONARY ARTERY TERRITORIES
Figure 7.13

Apical four-chamber (A4C) plane view and corresponding coronary artery territories and LV segments. Compare with Figures 2.9, 6.10, 6.23, 6.65, 7.36, 7.42.

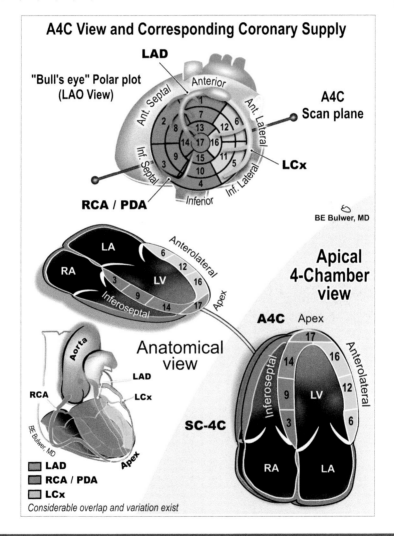

A4C: PHYSIOLOGY OF DIASTOLE
Figure 7.14

The cardiac cycle with emphasis on diastole. Echocardiography is an excellent tool for assessing several diastolic parameters: i). Left ventricular (LV) transmitral inflow Doppler, ii). Left atrial (LA) behavior and size, and iii). Mitral leaflet behavior. *AC: aortic valve closure; AO: aortic valve opening; MC: mitral valve closure; MO: mitral valve opening.*

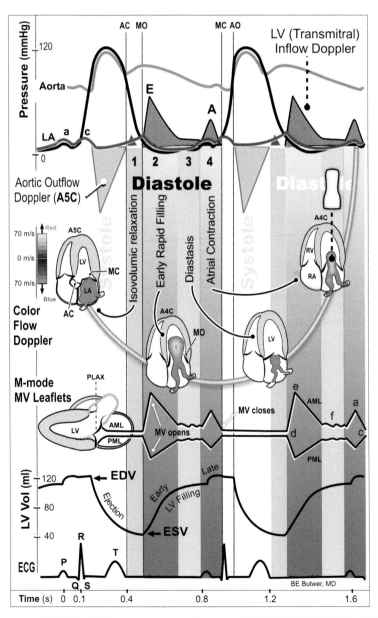

BE Bulwer, MD

A4C: LEFT ATRIAL DYNAMICS
Figure 7.15

Left atrial dynamics.

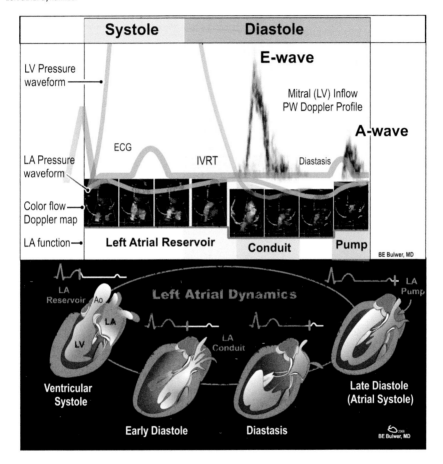

The atria exhibit dynamic behavior, both active and passive, during the cardiac cycle. They fill rapidly (and bulge) during systole, becoming smaller as they empty much of their blood into the left ventricle (LV) during diastole. The left atrium (LA) alternatively acts as a: (i) reservoir—receiving oxygenated blood from the lungs via the pulmonary veins during ventricular systole, (ii) conduit—(especially in early diastole) as blood empties into the left ventricle (LV), giving rise to the E wave on PW Doppler, and (iii) booster pump—with atrial contraction providing late diastolic LV filling, giving rise to the A wave on PW Doppler.

A4C: ASSESSMENT OF DIASTOLIC FUNCTION
Figure 7.16

Echocardiographic measures of diastole and diastolic dysfunction.

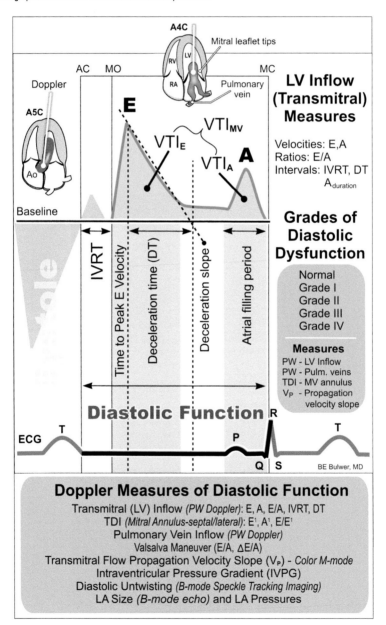

Doppler Measures of Diastolic Function
Transmitral (LV) Inflow *(PW Doppler)*: E, A, E/A, IVRT, DT
TDI *(Mitral Annulus-septal/lateral)*: E¹, A¹, E/E¹
Pulmonary Vein Inflow *(PW Doppler)*
Valsalva Maneuver (E/A, ΔE/A)
Transmitral Flow Propagation Velocity Slope (V$_P$) - *Color M-mode*
Intraventricular Pressure Gradient (IVPG)
Diastolic Untwisting *(B-mode Speckle Tracking Imaging)*
LA Size *(B-mode echo)* and LA Pressures

A4C: DIASTOLIC FUNCTION DOPPLER PARAMETERS AND GRADES OF DIASTOLIC DYSFUNCTION

Table 7.1 STAGES OF DIASTOLIC DYSFUNCTION

	Normal (young)	Normal (adult)	Delayed relaxation Grade I	Pseudonormal filling Grade II	Restrictive filling Grade III-IV
E/A	>1	>1	<1	1-2	>2
E DT (ms)	<220	<220	>220	150–200	<150
IVRT (ms)	<100	<100	>100	60–100	<60
Pulm. vein S/D	<1	≥1	≥1	<1	<1
Pulm. vein AR (cm/s)	<35	<35	<35	>35*	≥25*
E^1 (cm/sec), lateral mitral annulus	>12	>8–10	<8	<8	<8
LV relaxation	Normal	Normal	↓	↓	↓
LV filling pressure	Normal	Normal	↑	↑	↑

*Unless atrial mechanical failure present.
AR: pulmonary venous peak atrial contraction reversed velocity; **E^1:** early diastolic myocardial velocity on tissue Doppler imaging measured at the lateral mitral annulus; **E/A:** early-to-atrial left ventricular filling deceleration time; **E DT:** early left ventricular filling deceleration time; **IVRT:** isovolumic relaxation time; **S/D:** systolic-to-diastolic pulmonary venous flow ratio.

Reference: Adapted from Garcia MJ, Thomas JD, Klein AL. Doppler echocardiographic applications for the study of diastolic function. *J Am Coll Cardiol.* 1998;32:865–875.

Findings consistent with normal diastolic function

1. Normal transmitral LV inflow pattern with E:A ratio > 1.5 (on A4C view) with mitral deceleration time (DT) of 160–240 milliseconds in normal middle-aged adults. The deceleration slope should consider age (younger individuals have short DT due to rapid ventricular relaxation).
2. Normal pulmonary venous flow pattern with predominant diastolic flow that is with S:D ratio < 1 (on A4C view).
3. Normal tissue Doppler velocities measured at the mitral annulus (on A4C view).
4. Normal color M-mode flow propagation velocity with slope (VP) > 55 cm/sec.

A4C: PULMONARY VENOUS FLOW DOPPLER MEASUREMENT TECHNIQUE

Measuring Pulmonary Venous Flow (Figure 7.17)

1. From the apical 4-chamber view, using slight superior angulation (toward the aortic root), obtain optimal color flow Doppler-aided visualization of the pulmonary veins.
2. Using PW Doppler, place sample volume 1–2 cm into the pulmonary vein. The right-lower or upper-pulmonary vein is most optimally aligned for Doppler assessment in this view.
3. Sample from both pulmonary veins, and select whichever provides the best spectral pattern.
4. Adjust instrument settings, e.g., velocity filter, sample volume size, gain, or patient position as appropriate.

Figure 7.17

Measuring pulmonary venous flow.

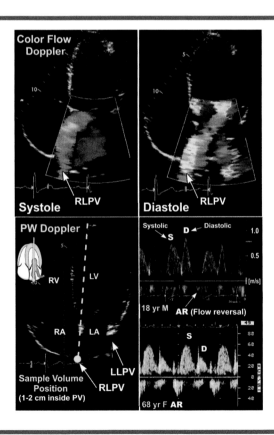

A4C: PULMONARY VENOUS FLOW DOPPLER ASSESSMENT
Figure 7.18

Pulmonary venous flow: normal vs. dysfunction. Doppler patterns of pulmonary venous flow. Abnormal pulmonary venous flow is characterized by blunting of the systolic wave and increased atrial reversal velocity and/or duration. *S: systolic flow; D: diastolic flow; AR: atrial reversal.*

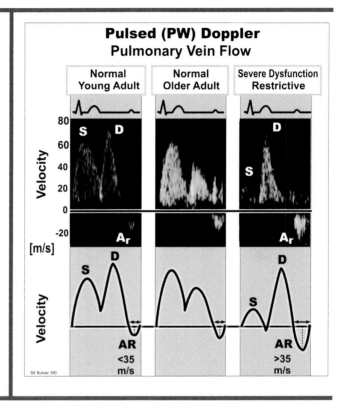

A4C: MEASUREMENT OF TRANSMITRAL LV INFLOW DOPPLER

Measurement of Left Ventricular (Transmitral) Inflow (Figure 7.19)

1. On the apical four-chamber (A4C) view, position PW Doppler sample volume at the tips of the mitral leaflets. (Flow at the annulus, or between the body of the leaflets, show lower peak velocities and shorter deceleration times than those obtained at the leaflet tips. E wave deceleration time lengthens when PW Doppler sample volume is too apically placed and shortens when the sample volume is too close to the mitral annulus.)

2. Align Doppler beam as parallel to flow as possible. Use color flow Doppler as a guide.

3. Adjust velocity scale according to the peak velocities recorded. (Normal range 60–130 cm/sec.)

4. Minimize velocity filters to record mid-diastolic flow, and eliminate wall motion artifacts.

5. Set sweep speed between 50 to 100 mm/sec.

6. Ask patient to breath-hold at end expiration, and record several cardiac cycles.

7. Analyze and correlate with other diastolic function measures Figures 7.16, 7.19 ; Table 7.1 .

Figure 7.19

Pulse wave (PW) Doppler profile of normal transmitral flow during diastole sampled at the tip of the mitral leaflets using the apical four-chamber (A4C) view. Note the early (E) and atrial contraction (A) velocities representing early and late diastolic filling. *DT: deceleration time.*

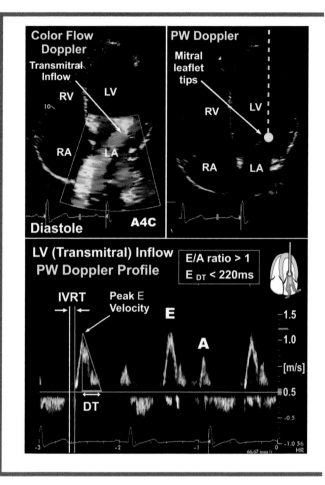

A4C: TRANSMITRAL LV INFLOW DOPPLER ASSESSMENT
Figure 7.20

Normal and abnormal transmitral LV inflow patterns and parameters seen in patients with progressive degrees of diastolic dysfunction.

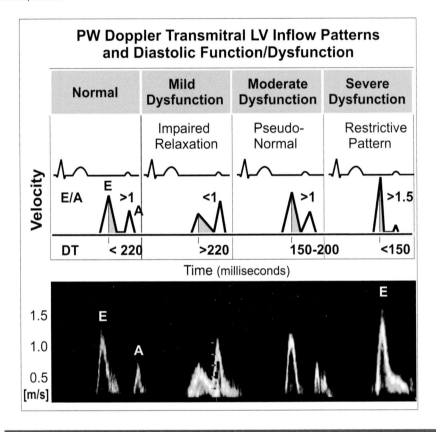

A4C: IVRT MEASUREMENT AND ASSESSMENT

Recording Isovolumetric Relaxation Time (IVRT) (Figure 7.21)

1. On the apical four-chamber (A4C) view using PW Doppler, position a 3–4 mm sample volume near the mitral leaflet tips to display mitral inflow. The transducer beam is then angulated toward the LV outflow tract until the transient of aortic valve closure appears above and below the baseline. IVRT is measured as the time interval between the aortic valve transient and the onset of mitral inflow.
2. If the results are suboptimal, CW Doppler can be used with similar positioning, to simultaneously record aortic and mitral flow. IVRT is measured as the time between the cessation of aortic flow and the onset of mitral flow.
3. Record the CW Doppler spectral profile.
4. Measure IVRT and correlate with other measures of LV function Figure 7.21 ; Table 7.1 .

Figure 7.21

Recording the isovolumetric relaxation time (IVRT). The isovolumetric relaxation time (IVRT) of the LV is the time interval between aortic valve closure (AC) to mitral valve opening (MO) and the start of transmitral flow (Figures 7.14, 7.16, 7.21). LA pressures and the rate of LV relaxation influence the IVRT. Excessive IVRT prolongation (>100 ms) is considered impaired relaxation. A shortened IVRT (<60 ms) is associated with elevation of LA pressure.

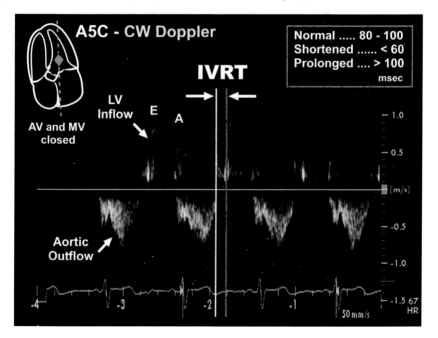

A4C: TISSUE DOPPLER IMAGING (TDI)

Optimal Doppler Tissue Imaging (DTI or TDI) Technique (Figures 4.24, 7.22, 7.23)

1. On the apical four-chamber (A4C) view, decrease the image depth (zoom) to visualize mitral annular region.
2. Set frame rate at 140–240 frames/second.
3. Set velocity scale 20:20.
4. Align tissue Doppler beam as parallel to the motion of the wall as possible.
5. Apply color tissue Doppler mode.
6. Place the sample volume at the ventricular side of the mitral annulus.
7. Set at the point where the ventricular wall remains within the sample volume during the cardiac cycle.
8. Use a sample volume of 3–6 mm. Use smaller sample volumes if LV systolic function is poor.
9. Optimize frame rate.
10. Apply PW tissue Doppler, ask patient to breath-hold, and at end-expiration.
11. Record several cycles.
12. Analyze TDI parameters of systolic and diastolic function, and correlate with other measures Figures 7.16, 7.22 ; Table 7.1 .

A4C: TISSUE DOPPLER IMAGING (TDI)
Figure 7.22

Recording the longitudinal mitral annular velocities on the apical 4-chamber view.

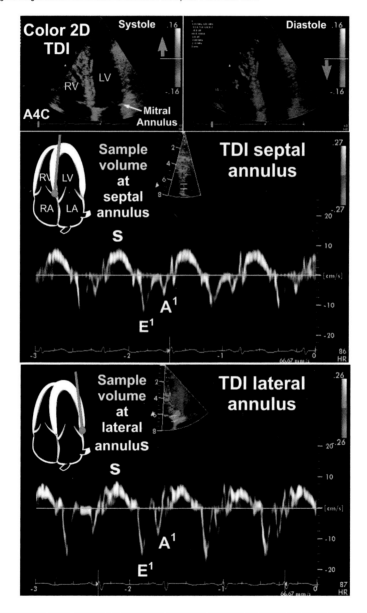

A4C VIEW: HOW TO MEASURE TDI
Figure 7.23

Doppler tissue imaging technique using the apical 4-chamber view.

Tissue Doppler Imaging (TDi) Technique

I. Apical 4-Chamber (A4C) View
Image at depths of 15 to 16 cm.
Ensure parallel Doppler beam alignment with the annulus to be assessed, i.e. septal or lateral.

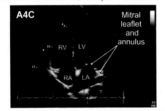

2. Decrease Depth
Decrease depth as shown, where the entire LV and less than half the atria are seen.

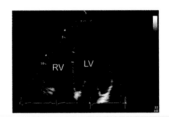

3. Activate Tissue Doppler
Activate TDI, DTI, or TVI - PW Doppler (according to manufacturer) at level of mitral annulus; Set velocity scale 20:20.

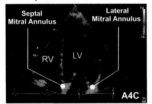

4. TDI Septal Mitral Annulus in A4C
PW Tissue Doppler at level of mitral annulus
Set velocity scale at 20:20
Adjust gain settings for optimal spectral display

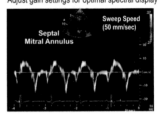

5. TDI to Septal Mitral Annulus (A4C)

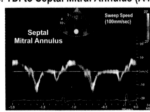

6. TDI to Lateral Mitral Annulus (A4C)

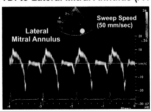

Repeat as in 4. (TDI septal annulus)

Common Pitfalls

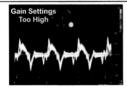

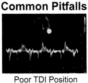

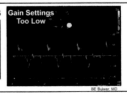

Poor TDI Position

BE Bulwer, MD

A4C: COMPOSITE MEASURES OF DIASTOLIC FUNCTION ASSESSMENT

Figure 7.24

Composite measures of diastolic dysfunction. Measures of diastolic function are best integrated with other parameters, including the wider clinical scenario (see Figure 7.16; Table 7.1).

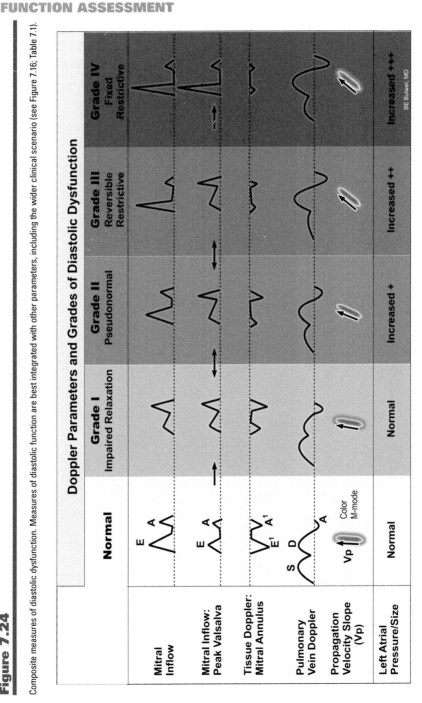

Figure 7.25

Color M-mode. The transmitral flow propagation velocity slope (Vp) assessed on the A4C view is another measure of LV diastolic performance. *Left.* Normal pattern with slope, Vp > 55cm/sec. *Right.* Abnormal flow propagation velocity with Vp < 55cm/sec.

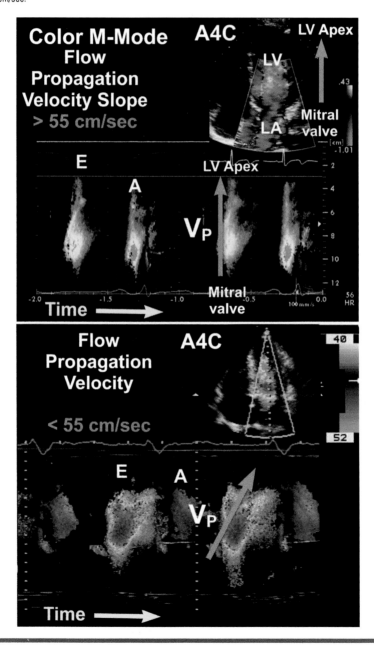

A4C VIEW: RV FUNCTION AND RV INFLOW
Figure 7.26

Tricuspid valve examination using color flow Doppler *(top)*, and CW Doppler *(bottom)* the apical four-chamber view (A4C). Compare TR velocities and derived indices with those obtained from the RV inflow view (Figure 6.41) and the PSAX-AVL view (Figure 6.55).

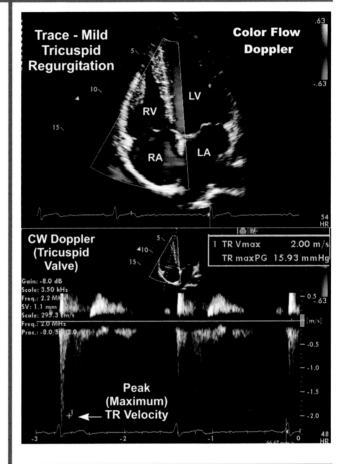

A4C VIEW: NORMAL AND ABNORMAL FINDINGS

Table 7.2 APICAL FOUR-CHAMBER (A4C) VIEW:
THE EXAMINATION SURVEY

Sequential survey	Findings: compare with findings in other views	
	Structural: on 2D, 3D, or M-mode	Functional and hemodynamic/ Doppler indices
Left atrium (LA)	Corroborate findings with the PLAX and PSAX views; see Tables 6.1, 6.5 MEASURE AND RECORD: by 2D and M-mode • LA size (systole) Figs. 6.12, 6.15 LA DIMENSIONS, AREAS, VOLUMES: Figs. 6.12, 6.15, 6.30 ; Table 12.6 LA CAVITY SIZE • Normal, increased, decreased • LA enlargement: mild, moderate, severe LA CAVITY APPEARANCE • Mass • "Smoke" (spontaneous echocontrast)	Corroborate findings with the PLAX and PSAX views; see Tables 6.1, 6.5 LA PHASIC DYNAMICS • LA acts as a "reservoir-conduit-pump" Figs. 7.14, 7.15 • Atrial fibrillation (loss of atrial "kick") • Spontaneous echocontrast "smoke" (best seen on TEE)
Mitral valve (MV)	Corroborate findings with the PLAX and PSAX views; see Tables 6.1, 6.5 MITRAL VALVE STRUCTURE Figs. 6.24, 6.61 • MV valves and supporting complex (chordae, papillary muscles, supporting LV wall/aorta) • Apical tenting of MV leaflets: in dilated cardiomyopathy • MV prolapse (MVP): MV is saddle shaped in the A4C view, so PLAX and A3C views are preferred for diagnosis of MVP • MS (thickened leaflets) • Infective endocarditis • MAC (mitral annular calcification), especially of posterior leaflet and annulus in the elderly • Prosthetic MV valve: mechanical vs. bioprosthetic	Corroborate findings with the PLAX and PSAX views; see Tables 6.1, 6.5 MITRAL REGURGITATION (MR) • Assess etiology • Estimate severity: mild, moderate, severe Fig. 6.25 MS SEVERITY ASSESSMENT • Assess etiology • Estimate severity: mild, moderate, severe Fig. 6.26 MV LEAFLET MOBILITY MITRAL VALVE SCORING CRITERIA IN mitral stenosis (MS) • Leaflet mobility • Subvalvular thickening • Valve leaflet thickening • Calcification

Table 7.2 APICAL FOUR-CHAMBER (A4C) VIEW:
THE EXAMINATION SURVEY *(continued)*

Sequential survey	Findings: compare with findings in other views	
	Structural: on 2D, 3D, or M-mode	Functional and hemodynamic/ Doppler indices
Left ventricle (LV)	LV CAVITY SIZE • LV enlargement (dilatation) Fig. 6.20 ; Table 12.1 • Decreased LV cavity size (volume depletion; also check IVC collapsibility index on subcostal view) Table 8.1 • Decreased LV cavity (due to cavity obliteration; markedly thickened walls) LV WALL THICKNESS Figs. 6.14, 6.15 • **LV hypertrophy** (≥12 mm in adults) including hypertrophic cardiomyopathy (most commonly asymmetric septal hypertrophy; discrete upper septal hypertrophy [DUSH]) LV WALL STRUCTURE • LV walls visualized and assessed: LV apex, anterolateral/lateral and inferoseptal/septal walls Figs. 6.21, 6.22, 7.8, 7.9, 7.13 • "Speckled" myocardium in infiltrative disease, e.g., amyloidosis • LV aneurysm or pseudoaneurysm, especially of posterior wall LV SEPTUM • VSD—membranous/ perimembranous • VSD (midseptal)—muscular (trabecular) LV MASSES • LV masses, e.g., thrombus, tumor • LV opacification using contrast agents often necessary LV DIMENSIONS, AREAS, VOLUMES Figs. 6.14, 6.15, 6.18–6.22 ; Tables 12.1–12.3	LV SYSTOLIC FUNCTION ASSESSMENT • Summary measures Figs. 6.18–6.23 LV WALL MOTION and WALL THICKENING • Wall motion score (WMS) and WMS index Figs. 6.21, 6.22 • Correlate with corresponding coronary artery blood supply Figs. 6.23, 7.8, 7.9, 7.13 LV EJECTION FRACTION • Figs. 6.18–6.20 ; Table 12.2 • "Eyeball estimate" of LV ejection fraction (LVEF) used in routine practice Figs. 6.19, 6.20 • Biplane method of disks (Simpson's rule) Fig. 6.20 LV DIASTOLIC FUNCTION Figs. 7.14–7.25 ; Table 7.1 • Doppler (pulmonary venous flow and S/D ratio)—A4C • Doppler (mitral inflow velocities and E/A ratio)—A4C • Doppler (isovolumetric relaxation time—IVRT)—A5C • Tissue Doppler imaging (TDI or DTI) • Color flow M-mode propagation velocity slope (Vp) • Enlarged left atrium: a feature of diastolic dysfunction

(continues)

Table 7.2 APICAL FOUR-CHAMBER (A4C) VIEW:
THE EXAMINATION SURVEY *(continued)*

Sequential survey	Findings: compare with findings in other views	
	Structural: on 2D, 3D, or M-mode	Functional and hemodynamic/ Doppler indices
Right atrium (RA)	RA CAVITY SIZE • Size: normal, increased, decreased • RA enlargement: mild, moderate, severe (note post cardiac transplant, cor triatriatum) RA CAVITY APPEARANCE • Mass—most commonly thrombus (clot), myxoma • Mass—Chiari network • Cardiac hardware • "Smoke" (spontaneous echocontrast) RA VIEWS • Fig. 6.44	RA PHASIC DYNAMICS • RA acts as "reservoir-conduit-pump" • Loss of atrial "pump" **(atrial fibrillation)** • Diastolic collapse of RA free wall—earliest sign in **pericardial tamponade** Fig. 6.33 ELEVATED RA PRESSURES (RAP) Figs. 4.5, 6.42 Signs of elevated RAP: • Dilated IVC with decreased respirophasic collapse—use subcostal-IVC view (see Fig. 8.9b ; Table 8.1) • Dilated tributary veins: IVC, SVC, coronary sinus • Dilated RA, RV • Severe TR • Bowing of interatrial septum toward the left (throughout cardiac cycle
Tricuspid valve (TV)	TV STRUCTURE • **Normal leaflet structure, mobility, thickness, and closure** (coaptation), chordae tendinae, papillary muscle • **Leaflet vegetation:** location, size, mobility TV LEAFLET MOBILITY • **Excessive movement of one or both leaflets:** prolapse, leaflet flail • **Restricted leaflet motion:** thickened immobile leaflets in carcinoid syndrome, rheumatic fever (rare) • Prosthetic MV: mechanical vs. bioprosthetic; normal vs. abnormal function; valve and paravalvular	TRICUSPID REGURGITATION (TR) • Peak velocity: CW Doppler • PASP (pulmonary artery systolic pressure) measurement (applying the Bernoulli equation to peak CW Doppler velocities). Add to right atrial pressure (RAP) estimates from IVC assessment (subcostal IVC view) Figs. 4.5, 6.40–6.42 • Assess etiology • Estimate severity: mild, moderate, severe Fig. 6.43a TRICUSPID STENOSIS (TS) • Assess etiology (carcinoid, rheumatic) • Estimate severity: mild, moderate, severe Fig. 6.43b

Table 7.2 APICAL FOUR-CHAMBER (A4C) VIEW:
THE EXAMINATION SURVEY *(continued)*

Sequential survey	Findings: compare with findings in other views	
	Structural: on 2D, 3D, or M-mode	Functional and hemodynamic/ Doppler indices
Right ventricle (RV)	RV/RVOT CAVITY • Dilatation, e.g., in pressure or volume overload states, e.g., right heart failure; primary and secondary pulmonary hypertension; secundum ASD Fig. 6.31 ; Tables 12.4, 12.5 • Pacemaker or defibrillator wire RV/RVOT WALL • Thickened in chronic overload states, e.g., chronic pulmonary hypertension	RV/RVOT CAVITY • Impaired contractility, e.g., in RV pressure and volume overload states RV/RVOT WALL • Diastolic collapse with pericardial effusion/tamponade—confirm on M-mode RV SYSTOLIC FUNCTION • "Eyeball" estimate of RV systolic function • RV diameters in systole and diastole • RV fractional area change
Pericardium	• Pericardial effusion • Pericardial thickening Corroborate findings with the PLAX view (see Table 6.1 ; Fig. 6.33)	• ± tamponade physiology • ± constrictive physiology Findings consistent with tamponade, including RV diastolic collapse
Coronary sinus (CS)	• Visible on A4C views at the level of the coronary sinus, or at the atrioventricular junction • Normal or dilated, as in persistent left superior vena cava (PLSVC) • Coronary sinus ASD	• Coronary sinus ASD: color flow Doppler (best views on TEE) • Contrast "bubble" study shows entry of contrast into coronary sinus before entering RA
Internal cardiac crux	• Normal crux Figs. 7.10, 7.11 • AV septal dysmorphology in atrioventricular canal (endocardial cushion) defects	Assess hemodynamic, regional, and global impact of atrioventricular canal defect

APICAL FIVE-CHAMBER (A5C) VIEW

The A5C view, also called the elevated A4C view, is used primarily to assess the left ventricular outflow tract (LVOT), the aortic valve (AV), and the aortic root (Ao) Figures 7.28–7.31 .

Patient and transducer positioning

The patient remains lying in the left lateral position, with superior angulation of the transducer to visualize the aortic valve and root Figures 7.1, 7.27, 7.28 .

Transducer maneuvers

From the A4C view, angulate the transducer scan plane cranially until the internal cardiac crux (atrioventriculo-valvular junction) is replaced by the LVOT, the AV, and aortic root Figures 7.28–7.30 .

2D scan sector image display

Identify, optimize, and record the structures shown in Figure 7.30 , including the LV, the LVOT, the aortic valve, aortic root, LA, and RV.

2D aortic valve examination 2D

Aortic valve (AV): Focus on the AV. Examine and assess valvular structures—annulus; cusps for mobility, thickening, calcification, or vegetations; commissures.

Doppler examination

- **Left ventricular outflow tract (LVOT)**→Color Doppler→PW Doppler Figures 7.17–7.18 ; Table 7.1 . PW Doppler interrogation along the interventricular septum from the apex to the valve can detect intracavitary gradients, including dynamic left ventricular outflow tract obstruction. In suspected or existing aortic stenosis, obtain PW Doppler measurement at approximately 1 cm below the aortic valve, i.e., within the LVOT.
- **Aortic valve (AV)**→Transmitral LV Inflow: Color Doppler→PW Doppler→CW Doppler→color M-mode (flow propagation velocity) Figures 7.14–7.16, 7.19–7.20 ; Table 7.1 . CW Doppler across the aortic valve detects peak transaortic gradients. Apply the freeze function and trace spectral Doppler envelope to quantify the velocity time integral (TVI or VTI). Perform CW Doppler across the aortic valve, and then measure TVI. From these, the aortic valve area can be calculated using continuity equation.

Coronary artery segments visualized on the PLAX view

Correlate abnormalities of ventricular wall motion and thickening with their corresponding coronary artery supply. These largely correlate with those of the A4C view Figures 2,9, 6.10, 6.23, 6.65, 7.13, 7.36, 7.42 .

Findings and Summaries

Assess cardiac structure and function. Confirm findings on complementary views Table 7.2 .

A5C: PATIENT POSITIONING AND TRANSDUCER PLACEMENT
Figure 7.27

The apical window and transducer orientation for obtaining the A5C view. Note the elevation required when starting from the A4C scan plane *(insert)*.

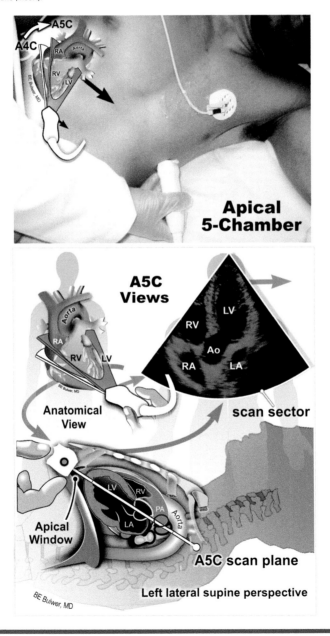

A5C: ANATOMICAL ORIENTATION
Figure 7.28

Anatomical projections of the apical five-chamber (A5C) scan plane *(left and center)*. The more widely used "apex-up" projection of the A5C view is shown above right. Compare with Figures 7.29 and 7.30.

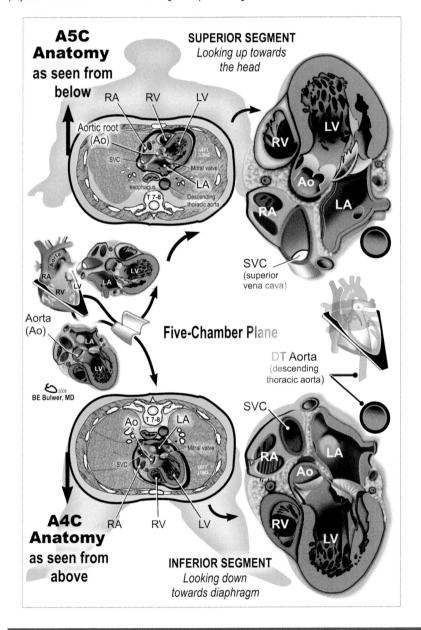

A5C: SCAN SECTOR ANATOMY
Figure 7.29

Apical five-chamber (A5C) views: scan plane and scan sector displays.

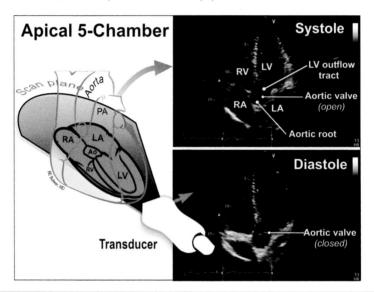

Figure 7.30

Diastolic still frame showing the cross-sectional anatomy of the apical five-chamber (A5C) view.

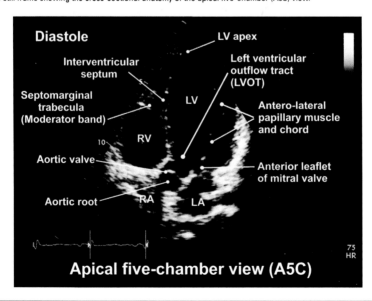

A5C: DOPPLER ASSESSMENT
Figure 7.31

Doppler examination of the apical five-chamber (A5C) view.

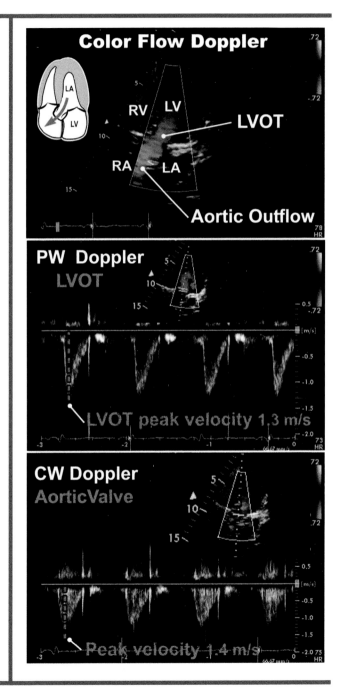

A5C SURVEY: NORMAL AND ABNORMAL FINDINGS
Table 7.3

Sequential Survey	Findings: Compare with findings in other views	
	Structural: on 2D, 3D, or M-Mode	Functional and Hemodynamic/Doppler Indices
Left Atrium (LA)	• Corroborate findings with the PLAX, A4C, and other views; see Tables 6.1, 7.2 • LA views and measures: Fig. 6.30 , Table 12.6	
Mitral Valve (MV)	• As for A4C: See Table 7.2 • MV scallops: Figs. 6.24, 6.61	• As for A4C: See Table 7.2 • Mitral regurgitation: Fig. 6.25 • Mitral stenosis: Fig. 6.26
Left Ventricle (LV)	• Corroborate findings with the PLAX, PSAX, A4C and other views: See Table 7.2 • Measures of LV structure and function: Figs. 6.18–6.23 , Tables 12.1–12.3	
LV Outflow Tract (LVOT)	LVOT OBSTRUCTION • Septal hypertrophy in hypertrophic cardiomyopathy (HCM) • Severe LV hypertrophy (LVH) • Systolic anterior motion (SAM) of the anterior mitral valve leaflet in HCM • Discrete upper septal hypertrophy (DUSH) • Subvalvular membrane	DOPPLER ASSESSMENT • Color flow, PW, and CW Doppler: for signs of accelerated flow with SAM or subvalvular membrane. • Measure LVOT diameter 1cm proximal to AV leaflets (for calculation of stroke volume/cardiac output or for aortic valve area calculation in aortic stenosis (AS)) Figs. 4.15, 6.27, 6.29
Aortic Valve (AV)	AV STRUCTURE Figs. 6.9, 6.12, 6.27, 6.29 • Observe the normal trileaflet (cusps) structure identify: leaflets, annulus, sinus of Valsalva, aortic root • **Thickened and echoreflective "calcified" AV leaflets ± annulus** in aortic sclerosis (elderly), aortic stenosis (AS) • **valvular thickening and systolic doming** with bicuspid aortic valve (BAV); quadricuspid and unicuspid variants • Aortic dimensions Fig. 6.27 • **Mobile** vegetation(s) ± leaflet perforation in infective endocarditis, papillary fibroelastoma, Lambl's excrescences. • Prosthetic AV valve: mechanical vs. bioprosthetic • **Supravalvular thickening**	AORTIC REGURGITATION (AR): • Assess etiology • Estimate severity: mild, moderate, severe Fig. 6.28 AORTIC STENOSIS (AS) • Assess etiology • Estimate severity: mild, moderate, severe Figs. 4.15, 6.29, 10.2 AORTIC DISSECTION (AD): • Color flow Doppler and spectral Doppler: new onset AR (with aortic root dissection) • ± Pericardial tamponade physiology (Doppler findings) AORTIC ANEURYSMS: Aortic root, ascending, arch, descending thoracic, abdominal • ± Aortic regurgitation (AR) with Doppler findings

Table 7.3 (continued)

Sequential Survey	Findings: Compare with findings in other views	
	Structural: on 2D, 3D, or M-Mode	Functional and Hemodynamic/ Doppler Indices
	MEASURE AND RECORD: by 2D and M-mode `Fig. 6.27` • **Aortic diameters** at various levels: aortic annulus, sinus of Valsalva	
Aortic Root (Ao)	• Aortic root dilatation: in hypertension, Marfan syndrome, bicuspid aortic valve disease (BAV) • Sinus of Valsalva aneurysm • Intimal flap (aortic dissection) in aortic root or ascending aorta ± aortic leaflet prolapse (new onset AR) • MEASURE AND RECORD: `Fig. 6.27` **Aortic diameters** at aortic annulus, sinus of Valsalva	AORTIC ANEURYSMS: Aortic root, ascending, arch, descending thoracic, abdominal • ± Aortic regurgitation (AR) with Doppler findings SUPRAVALVULAR AORTIC STENOSIS (AS): • Assess etiology • Estimate severity: mild, moderate, severe AORTIC DISSECTION (AD): • Color flow Doppler and spectral Doppler: new onset AR (with aortic root dissection) • ± Pericardial tamponade physiology (Doppler)
Right ventricle (RV)	• Corroborate findings with the PLAX, RV Inflow, A4C, and other views; see `Tables 6.1, 7.2`; RV Views `Figs. 6.31, 6.32`	
Pericardium	• Pericardial effusion • Pericardial thickening	• ± tamponade physiology • ± constrictive physiology

APICAL TWO-CHAMBER (A2C) VIEW

The A2C view, also called the vertical long-axis view, is used primarily to assess the LV apex, the anterior and inferior walls of the left ventricle (LV), the mitral valve (MV), and left atrium (LA) and atrial appendage (LAA) Figures 7.32–7.37 . As the A2C plane is considered orthogonal to the A4C plane, it is used in biplane Simpson's method for calculating LV volumes Figure 6.40 .

Patient and transducer positioning

The patient remains lying in the left lateral position, with the transducer scan plane oriented vertically, from the LV apex toward the neck Figures 7.32, 7.33 .

Transducer maneuvers

From the A4C view (with the transducer at ~3 o'clock position), rotate the transducer scan plane ~ 90° anticlockwise until the right-sided structures—the RA, RV, and TV—disappear, with the left-sided structures remaining in focus. Ensure that the LV long axis is vertically aligned, i.e., with the minimum Doppler angle, within the scan sector. Avoid excessive rotation toward the right shoulder (A3C view); this would encompass the LV outflow tract and aortic root Figures 7.1, 7.32–7.34 .

2D scan sector image display

Identify, optimize, and record the anterior and inferior walls of the LV—the surface that sits on the diaphragm, the mitral valve, left atrium (LA), and appendage, the coronary sinus (CS) in the atrioventricular groove. Identify, optimize, and record structures shown in Figures 7.34 and 7.35 .

Assess and measure LV and LA chamber size and function, including the biplane Simpson's method Figures 6.18–6.23, 6.30 ; Tables 12.1–12.3, 12.6 .

Doppler examination

- **Mitral valve (MV)**→Transmitral LV Inflow: Color Doppler→PW Doppler→CW Doppler→ Figures 7.14–7.16, 7.19–7.20 ; Table 7.1 .
- **Mitral annulus (septal and lateral)**→Tissue Doppler Imaging of mitral annular (longitudinal) velocities Figure 7.37 , see Figures 7.22, 7.23 ; Table 7.1 .

Coronary artery segments visualized on the PLAX view

Correlate abnormalities of ventricular wall motion and thickening with their corresponding coronary artery supply Figures 2.9, 6.10, 6.23, 6.65, 7.13, 7.36, 7.42 .

Findings and Summaries

Assess cardiac structure and function. Confirm findings on complementary views Table 7.4 .

A2C: PATIENT POSITIONING AND TRANSDUCER PLACEMENT
Figure 7.32

View of the apical window and transducer orientation for obtaining A2C views. Note the direction of the transducer index mark (black arrow) and the transducer maneuvers. Compare with Figures 7.4–7.6.

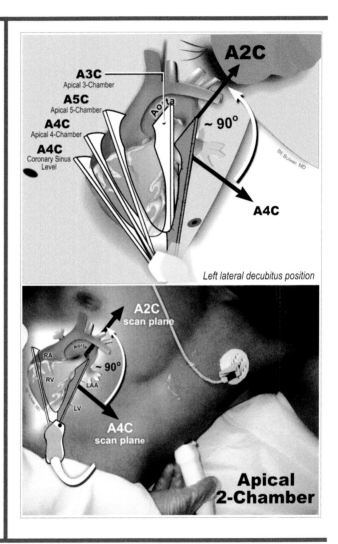

APICAL 2-CHAMBER SCAN PLANES, ANATOMY, AND SCAN SECTOR DISPLAY
Figure 7.33

Panoramic perspectives of the apical two-chamber (A2C) view scan plane, scan plane anatomy, and image display.

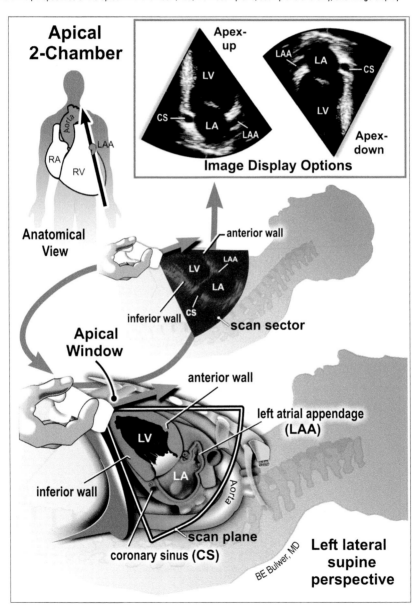

A2C: SCAN SECTOR ANATOMY
Figure 7.34

The apical two-chamber (A2C): scan plane and scan sector displays.

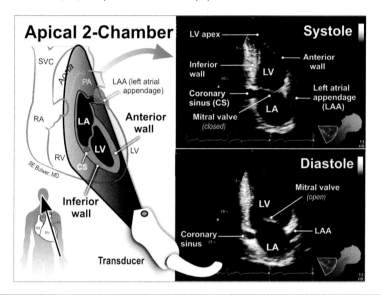

Figure 7.35

Systolic still frame showing the cross-sectional anatomy of the apical two-chamber (A2C) view.

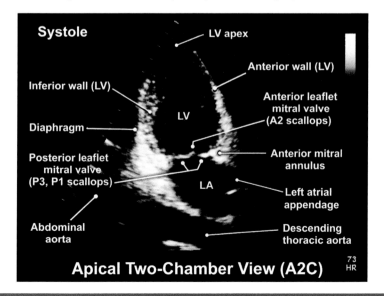

A2C VIEW AND CORONARY ARTERY TERRITORIES
Figure 7.36

The apical two-chamber (A2C) view and corresponding coronary artery territories and LV segments. Compare with Figures 2.9, 6.10, 6.23, 7.13, 7.42.

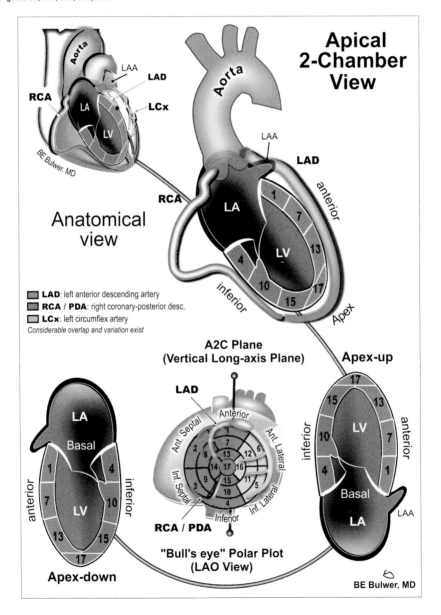

Apical 2-Chamber View

LAA
LAD
RCA
LA
LV
LCx
BE Bulwer, MD

Aorta

Anatomical view

LAA
LAD
RCA
LA
LV
anterior
inferior
Apex

1 7 13 4 10 17 15

LAD: left anterior descending artery
RCA / PDA: right coronary-posterior desc.
LCx: left circumflex artery
Considerable overlap and variation exist

**A2C Plane
(Vertical Long-axis Plane)**

Apex-up

LAD
Anterior
Ant. Septal
Ant. Lateral
Inf. Septal
Inf. Lateral
Inferior
RCA / PDA

**"Bull's eye" Polar Plot
(LAO View)**

1 2 8 7 13 12 6 14 17 16 9 15 10 11 3 5 4

LA
Basal
anterior
inferior
LV
1 4 7 10 13 15 17
Apex-down

17 15 13 10 LV 7 4 1
inferior
anterior
Basal
LA
LAA

BE Bulwer, MD

A2C: DOPPLER ASSESSMENT
Figure 7.37

Apical long-axis or apical two-chamber (A2C) view.

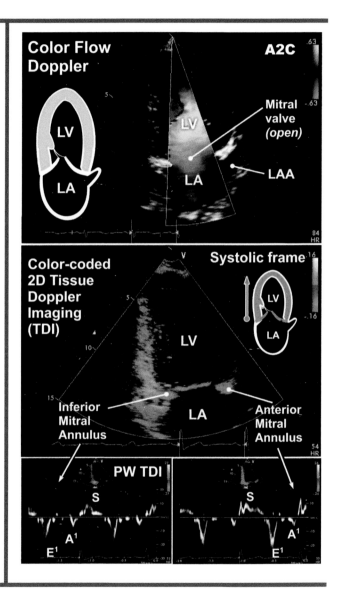

A2C SURVEY: NORMAL AND ABNORMAL FINDINGS

Table 7.4 APICAL TWO-CHAMBER (A2C) VIEW: THE EXAMINATION SURVEY

Sequential survey	*Findings: compare with findings in* other views	
	Structural: on 2D, 3D, or M-Mode	Functional and hemodynamic/ Doppler indices
Left atrium (LA)	• Corroborate findings with the PLAX, A4C, and other views; see Tables 6.1, 7.2 ; Fig. 6.30	
Mitral valve (MV)	• As for PLAX and A4C views: see Tables 6.1, 7.2 • Note leaflet scallops Figs. 6.24, 6.61	• As for PLAX and A4C views: See Tables 6.1, 7.2 • Mitral regurgitation Fig. 6.25 • Mitral stenosis Fig. 6.26
Left ventricle (LV)	• As for A4C: See Table 7.2 • Fig. 6.20 , Table 12.1 LV WALL STRUCTURE: LV APEX, ANTERIOR, and INFERIOR WALLS • LV walls visualized and assessed: Figs. 6.21, 6,22, 7.34–7.36 • LV hypertrophy including hypertrophic cardiomyopathy (HCM) • Papillary muscle: displacement, rupture • LV wall aneurysm, pseudoaneurysm	As for A4C: See Table 7.2 LV WALL MOTION LV APEX, ANTERIOR, and INFERIOR WALLS • Wall Motion Score (WMS) and WMS Index Figs. 6.21, 6.22 . • Correlate with corresponding coronary artery blood supply Figs. 6.23, 7.34–7.36 LV EJECTION FRACTION • Figs. 6.18–6.20 , Table 12.2 . • "Eyeball estimate" of LV ejection fraction (LVEF) used in routine practice Figs. 6.19, 6.20 • Biplane method of disks (Simpson's rule) Fig. 6.20 LV DIASTOLIC FUNCTION Figs. 7.14–7.25 ; Table 7.1 • Tissue Doppler Imaging (TDI) to MV annulus • Color flow M-mode
Pericardium	• Pericardial effusion • Pericardial thickening	• ± tamponade physiology • ± constrictive physiology
Descending thoracic aorta (DTAo)	• Long-axis view of the descending thoracic aorta (DTAo) often seen Figs. 6.27, 7.35 , but image resolution often suboptimal; best assessed by transesophageal echocardiography (TEE) • Intimal flap of aortic dissection (AD) in the DTAo may be evident	• Color flow Doppler: Differential color flow velocities DTAo—in the true and false lumen may be evident in aortic dissection (AD)

APICAL THREE-CHAMBER (A3C) VIEW

The A3C view, also called the apical long-axis (ALAX) view, is aligned parallel to the long-axis plane like the parasternal long-axis (PLAX) view. Unlike the PLAX view, the A3C scan plane transects the LV apex and apical segments. It is used to assess the LV apex, anteroseptal, and inferolateral ("posterior") walls of the left ventricle (LV), left ventricular outflow tract (LVOT), aortic root (Ao), the mitral valve (MV), and left atrium (LA) [Figures 7.38–7.43].

Patient and transducer positioning

The patient remains lying in the left lateral position, with the transducer scan plane oriented toward the right shoulder [Figures 7.38, 7.39].

Transducer maneuvers

Maneuvering from the A2C scan plane (with the index mark toward the neck) to the A3C scan plane (with the index mark pointing toward the right shoulder) requires further anticlockwise rotation of ~45° when starting from the A4C scan plane [Figures 7.38, 7.39].

2D scan sector image display

Identify, optimize, and record structures shown in [Figures 7.39–7.41].

Assess and measure LV and LA chamber size and function, including the biplane Simpson's method [Figures 6.18–6.23, 6.30]; [Tables 12.1–12.3, 12.6].

Doppler Examination sequence: The A3C view can be used to complement Doppler examination of the LVOT and the AV.

- **Left ventricular outflow tract (LVOT)** → Color Doppler→PW Doppler [Figures 7.17–7.18]; [Table 7.1]. PW Doppler interrogation along the interventricular septum from the apex to the valve can detect intracavitary gradients, including dynamic left ventricular outflow tract obstruction. In suspected or existing aortic stenosis, obtain PW Doppler measurement at approximately 1 cm below the aortic valve, i.e., within the LVOT.
- **Aortic valve (AV)**→Transmitral LV Inflow: Color Doppler→PW Doppler→CW Doppler→color M-mode (flow propagation velocity) [Figures 7.14–7.16, 7.19–7.20]; [Table 7.1]. CW Doppler across the aortic valve detects peak transaortic gradients. Apply the freeze function and trace spectral Doppler envelope to quantify the velocity time integral (TVI or VTI). Perform CW Doppler across the aortic valve and then measure TVI. From these, the aortic valve area can be calculated using continuity equation.
- **Mitral valve (MV)**→Transmitral LV Inflow: Color Doppler→PW Doppler→CW Doppler→color M [Figures 7.14–7.16, 7.19–7.20]; [Table 7.1].

Coronary artery segments visualized on the PLAX view

Correlate abnormalities of ventricular wall motion and thickening with their corresponding coronary artery supply Figures 2.9, 6.10, 6.23, 6.65, 7.13 .

Findings and Summaries

Assess cardiac structure and function. Confirm findings on complementary views Table 7.2 .

A3C: PATIENT POSITIONING AND TRANSDUCER PLACEMENT
Figure 7.38

Patient and transducer positioning: apical long-axis (apical three-chamber [A3C] view).

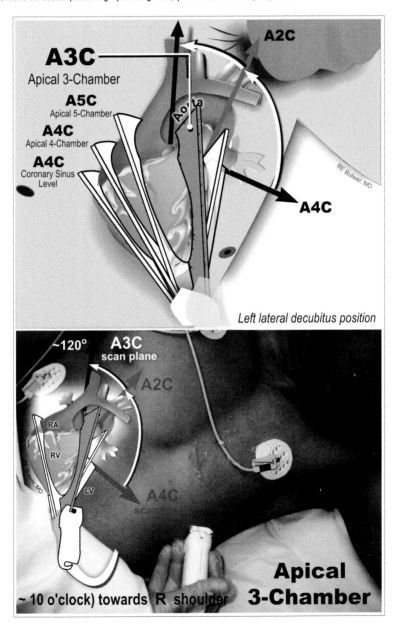

APICAL 3-CHAMBER SCAN PLANES, ANATOMY, AND SCAN SECTOR DISPLAY
Figure 7.39

Panoramic perspectives of the apical three-chamber (A3C) view scan plane, scan plane anatomy, and image display.

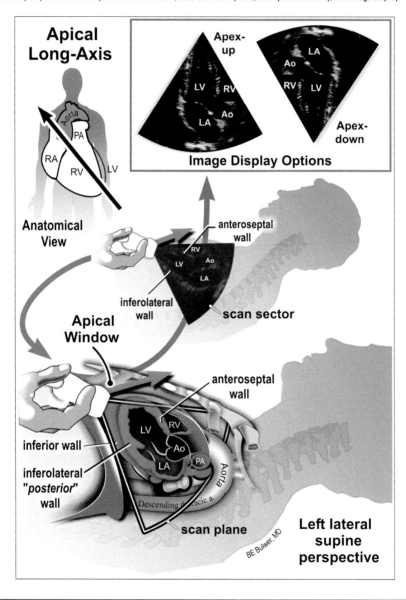

A5C: SCAN SECTOR ANATOMY
Figure 7.40

Apical long-axis or apical three-chamber (AC3) view and image display using the ASE recommended apex-up projection. This displays the RV on the right of the image display.

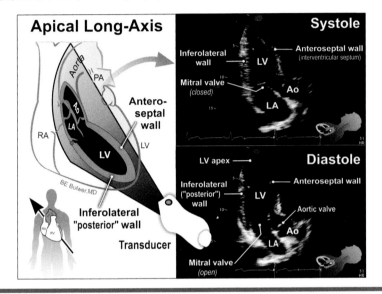

Figure 7.41

Systolic still frame showing the cross-sectional anatomy of the apical three-chamber (A3C) view.

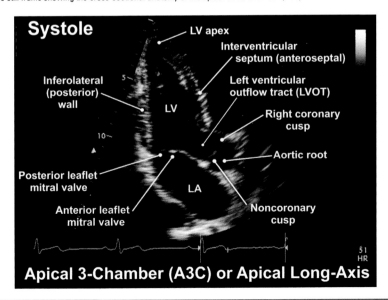

A3C VIEW AND CORONARY ARTERY TERRITORIES
Figure 7.42

The apical three-chamber (A3C) view and corresponding coronary artery territories and LV segments. Compare with Figures 2.9, 6.10, 6.23 7.13, 7.36. The parasternal long-axis (PLAX) view and the apical long-axis (ALAX, or apical three-chamber, A3C) views visualize the same LV segments. However, in the PLAX view, the LV apex and LV apical segments are not visualized.

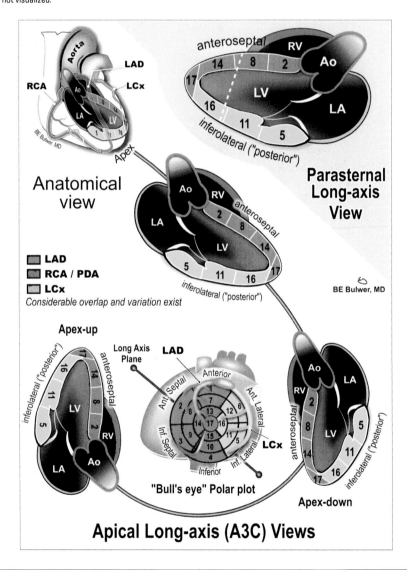

Apical Long-axis (A3C) Views

A3C: DOPPLER ASSESSMENT
Figure 7.43

Color flow Doppler examination of the apical three-chamber (A3C) views. *Upper panel.* Diastolic frame shows red flow velocities moving from the left atrium (LA) toward the left ventricle (LV). *Lower panel.* Systolic frame shows blue flow velocities moving from left ventricle (LV), the left ventricular outflow tract, and into the aortic root and ascending aorta (Ao).

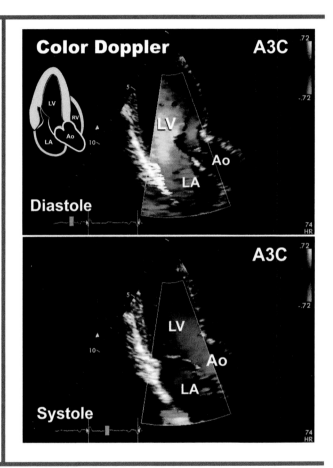

A3C SURVEY: NORMAL AND ABNORMAL FINDINGS

Table 7.5 APICAL THREE-CHAMBER (A3C) VIEW: THE EXAMINATION SURVEY

Sequential survey	Findings: compare with findings in other views	
	Structural: on 2D, 3D, or M-Mode	Functional and hemodynamic/ Doppler indices
LA	• As for PLAX and A4C views: See Tables 6.1, 7.2, 12.6 ; Fig. 6.30	
Mitral Valve	• As for PLAX and A4C views: See Tables 6.1, 7.2 • Note leaflet scallops Figs. 6.24, 6.61	• As for PLAX and A4C views: See Tables 6.1, 7.2 • Mitral regurgitation Fig. 6.25 • Mitral stenosis Fig. 6.26
LV	• As for A4C: See Table 7.2 • Fig. 6.20 , Table 12.1 LV wall structure: LV apex, anteroseptal, and inferolateral (or "posterior") walls • LV walls visualized and assessed: Figs. 6.21, 6.22, 7.34–7.36 • LV hypertrophy, including hypertrophic cardiomyopathy (HCM) • Papillary muscle: displacement, rupture • LV wall aneurysm, pseudoaneurysm	• As for A4C: See Table 7.2 LV wall motion and thickening: LV apex, anteroseptal, and infero-lateral (or "posterior") walls • Wall Motion Score (WMS) and WMS Index Figs. 6.21, 6.22 . • Correlate with corresponding coronary artery blood supply Figs. 6.23, 7.34–7.36
Aortic valve, aortic root; ascending aorta (Ao)	• Corroborate findings with the PLAX, A4C, and other views; see Tables 6.1, 7.2 • Aortic views: Fig. 6.27	
RV	• Corroborate findings with the PLAX, RV Inflow, A4C, and other views; see Tables 6.1, 7.2 ; RV Views Figs. 6.31, 6.32	
Pericardium	• Pericardial effusion • Pericardial thickening	• ± Tamponade physiology • ± Constrictive physiology

CHAPTER 8

Subcostal Windows and Views

In the comprehensive adult examination protocol Table 5.4 ; Figure 5.4 , the sub-costal window is primarily used to complement the parasternal and apical views, as well as to record long-axis views of the inferior vena cava (IVC), hepatic veins (Hv), and the proximal abdominal aorta (AA). Right-sided cardiac structures, particularly the right atrium (RA), interatrial septum (IAS), and right ventricle (RV), can be optimally examined because of their proximity and perpendicular orientation to the transducer scan plane.

In patients with obstructive lung diseases like emphysema, and where chest wall pathology or procedures render the parasternal and apical windows inacces-sible, a complete examination with corresponding long- and short-axis views can be obtained from the subcostal window Figures 8.5–8.8 .

In pediatric echocardiography, the subcostal (subxiphoid) window is where the examination begins. The sequential segmental analysis, which involves deter-mination of abdominal situs (site or location) and cardiac segments in patients with congenital heart disease, is readily established by the subxiphoid examina-tion Figure 6.69 ; Table 8.2 .

Patient and transducer positioning

The subcostal examination is best performed with the patient supine with the knees flexed Figures 8.1, 8.2 . The knee-flexed position relaxes the muscles of the anterior abdominal wall, thereby facilitating transducer placement and maneu-vers. Breath holding at end-inspiration moves the diaphragm downward, thereby moving the heart closer to the transducer. Gently but firmly position the trans-ducer (with acoustic coupling gel) in the upper-epigastric region, just below the xiphoid process (xiphisternum) while directing the scan plane toward the in-tended target, and with the appropriate transducer maneuvers.

Transducer maneuvers, scan plane orientation, and anatomy

To perform the subcostal long-axis sweep Figures 8.5, 8.6 , also called the sub-costal four-chamber or coronal sweep, scan from the inferior surface of the heart that sits on the diaphragm (coronary sinus plane), along an arc that sweeps through the four-chamber (SC-4C) plane, the long-axis plane of the left ventric-ular outflow tract (LVOT), and the long-axis plane of the right ventricular outflow tract (RVOT). Identify, optimize, and record the structures shown, followed by Doppler interrogation of specific regions of interest.

In the comprehensive examination, only the subcostal four-chamber (SC-4C) view is routinely recorded. For this view, hold the transducer as shown Figures 8.1, 8.2 , with the transducer pointing toward the left shoulder (but under the ribs), and index mark pointing toward the left loin (~3 to 5 o'clock) position. Identify, optimize, and record the structures shown in Figures 8.3, 8.4, 8.8 .

To perform the subcostal short-axis sweep Figure 8.7 , rotate 90° anticlockwise from the long-axis plane, scanning from right to left, sweep from the level of the cardiac apex, through the mid-LV level, through to the cardiac base, the aorta, and finally toward the RA as it receives the superior and inferior vena cavae. Identify, optimize, and record the structures shown, followed by Doppler interrogation of specific regions of interest.

SUBCOSTAL 4-CHAMBER VIEWS: PATIENT POSITIONING AND TRANSDUCER

Figure 8.1

Patient and transducer positioning: subcostal window: patient supine with knees flexed.

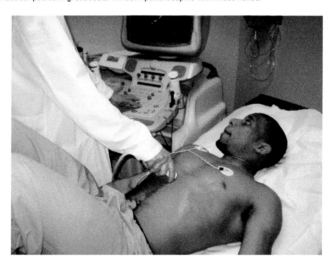

Figure 8.2

Patient and transducer positioning: subcostal window. Note the position of the index mark (dot) at approximately the 3 to 4 o'clock position. Note also generous amounts of acoustic coupling gel applied to promote optimal ultrasound transmission.

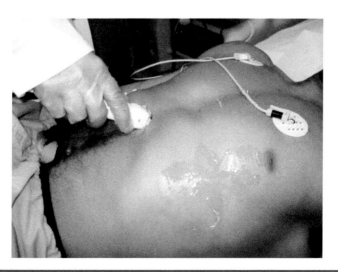

SUBCOSTAL FOUR-CHAMBER (SC-4C) VIEW

2D scan sector image display

Using the transducer maneuvers described previously, identify, optimize, record, and assess the structures shown in ⟨ Figures 8.4, 8.8 ⟩. The SC-4C view provides superior visualization of the interatrial septum (IAS), right ventricle (RV), right atrium (RA), and interventricular septum, in addition to the four-cardiac chambers. Morphologic criteria of the cardiac chambers can be performed using this view ⟨ Table 8.2 ⟩.

M-mode

When indicated, e.g., in the clinical setting of a pericardial effusion and suspected pericardial tamponade, M-mode examination can confirm the timing of abnormal wall motion of the cardiac chambers and interventricular septum (IVS), e.g., diastolic collapse of the free wall of the RA and RV, as well as abnormal septal movements.

DOPPLER EXAMINATION

- Interatrial septum (IAS): Interrogate IAS for possible patent foramen ovale (PFO) or atrial septal defect (ASD) using color flow Doppler. Apply PW Doppler when indicated ⟨ Figure 8.9b ⟩; ⟨ Table 8.3 ⟩.
- Mitral valve (MV), Tricuspid valve (TV), Interventricular septum (IVS): Apply color flow Doppler ⟨ Figure 8.9a ⟩.

Coronary artery segments visualized on the PLAX view

Correlate abnormalities of ventricular wall motion and thickening with their corresponding coronary artery supply. These segments largely correspond to those obtained on the apical four-chamber view ⟨ Figures 2.9, 6.10, 6.23, 6.65, 7.13 ⟩.

Findings and Summaries

Assess cardiac structure and function. Confirm findings on complementary views ⟨ Table 7.2 ⟩.

SC-4C SCAN PLANES, ANATOMY, AND SCAN SECTOR DISPLAY
Figure 8.3

Subcostal four-chamber (SC-4C) view: scan plane and anatomical perspectives.

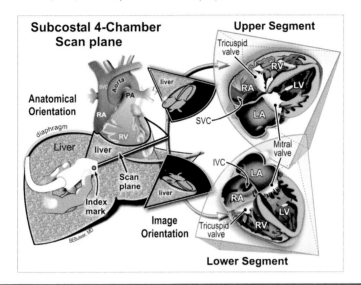

Figure 8.4

Subcostal four-chamber (SC-4C) view: cross-sectional anatomy.

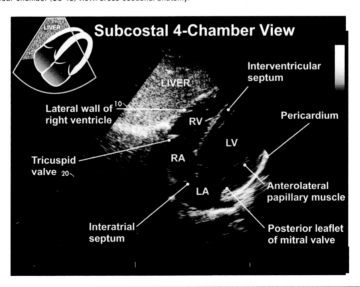

SUBCOSTAL LONG-AXIS "SWEEP" SCAN PLANES—LATERAL ANATOMICAL PERSPECTIVES
Figure 8.5

Left lateral supine perspective of the subcostal four-chamber and outflow tract views. *PA: main pulmonary artery; LA: left atrium; LV: left ventricle; RV: right ventricle.*

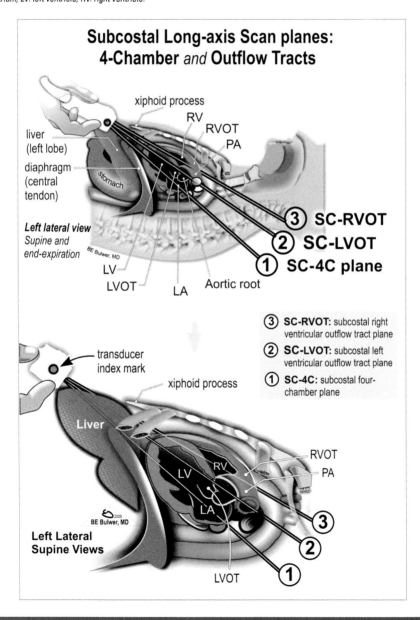

SUBCOSTAL LONG-AXIS "SWEEP" SCAN PLANES—
ANATOMICAL VIEWS
Figure 8.6

Subxiphoid (subcostal) long-axis scan planes and related cardiac anatomy visualized on the examination. *IVC: inferior vena cava; LV: left ventricle; MV: mitral valve; PA: pulmonary artery; RV: right ventricle; RPA: right pulmonary artery; SVC: superior vena cava; TV: tricuspid valve.*

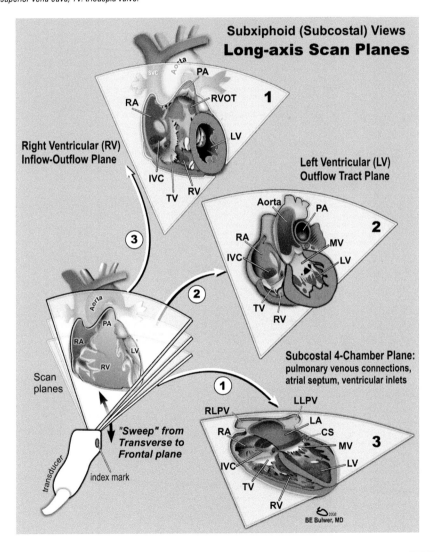

SUBCOSTAL SHORT-AXIS "SWEEP" SCAN PLANES— ANATOMICAL VIEWS

Figure 8.7

Subxiphoid (subcostal) short-axis scan planes "sweep," image projections, and related cardiac anatomy visualized on the pediatric echocardiographic examination. *IVC: inferior vena cava; LV: left ventricle; MV: mitral valve; PA: pulmonary artery; RV: right ventricle; RPA: right pulmonary artery; SVC: superior vena cava; TV: tricuspid valve.*

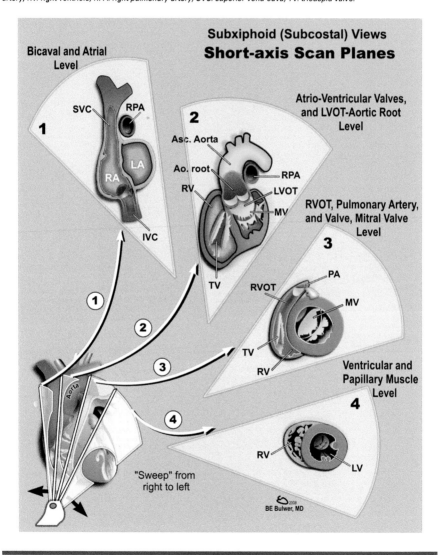

SC-4C, INFERIOR VENA CAVA, AND ABDOMINAL AORTA: SCAN PLANES AND SCAN SECTOR

Figure 8.8

Subcostal four-chamber view (SC-4C). Anatomy, scan planes, and image displays.

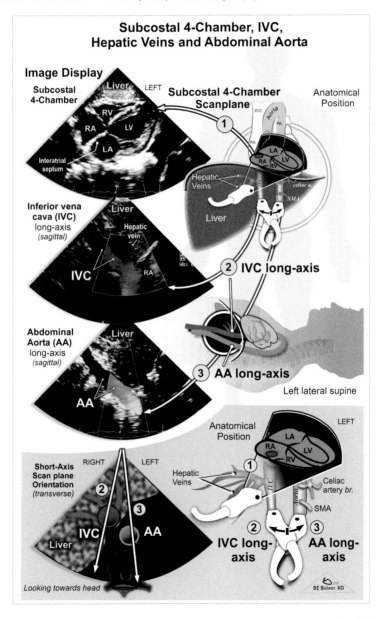

SC-4C AND INFERIOR VENA CAVA: DOPPLER EXAMINATION
Figure 8.9a

Above. Color flow Doppler examination of the subcostal four-chamber (SC-4C) view. This view provides optimal imaging of the interatrial septum (IAS) due to its perpendicular orientation to the ultrasound scan plane. Interrogation of the IAS by color Doppler can reveal a patent foramen ovale (PFO) or an atrial septal defect (ASD). Color flow Doppler can also assess the interventricular septum and atrioventricular valves. *Below.* Zoomed view of the interatrial septum reveals flow convergence at the left atrial side of a secundum-type ASD. Note the red color jet, which is indicative of left-to-right flow across the ASD and toward the transducer.

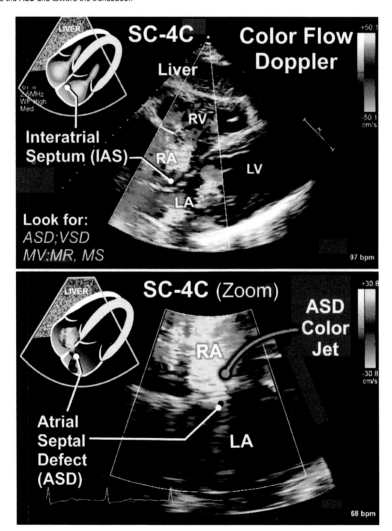

SUBCOSTAL IVC LONG-AXIS (SC-IVC-LAX) VIEW

Examination of the inferior vena cava (IVC) and its tributary hepatic veins allows the assessment of parameters central to the noninvasive assessment of intracardiac hemodynamics—specifically right atrial (RA) pressures `Table 8.1`; see `Figures 4.5, 6.42`. The IVC size and its respirophasic dynamics are used to estimate RA pressures (RAP). The RAP, in conjunction with the pressure gradient derived from the peak tricuspid regurgitant jet velocity, is used to estimate pulmonary artery systolic pressure (PASP) `Figures 4.5, 6.41, 6.42`.

Patient and transducer positioning

Patient's position remains the same as for the previous subcostal examination of the heart—that is, with the patient supine and the knees flexed `Figures 8.1, 8.2`.

Transducer maneuvers and scan plane orientation

To examine the subcostal long axis of the inferior vena cava (SC-IVC LAX) from the SC-4C view, rotate the scan plane 90° anticlockwise, while keeping the RA in view until aligned as shown in `Figures 8.8, 8.9b`. The index mark should be at ~ the 12 o'clock position. Ensure visualization of the IVC as it enters the R atrium. This helps to avoid mistaking the aorta for the IVC. Note that the abdominal aorta has a thicker (hyperechoic) wall and exhibits visible pulsations. Interrogation with color flow Doppler and PW Doppler readily distinguishes the two `Figures 8.8, 8.9b, 8.10`.

2D scan sector image display

Identify, optimize, and record the liver and intrahepatic veins as they enter into the IVC `Figures 8.8, 8.9b`. Optimize the long axis of the IVC as it enters into the right atrium (RA). Measure IVC diameter and observe its respirophasic behavior and use to estimate RAP `Table 8.1`; see `Figures 4.5, 6.42`. Measure the IVC diameter at 1 to 2 cm from the IVC-RA junction. Ensure that the IVC diameter is measured perpendicular to the IVC long axis. Note that the IVC diameter decreases with inspiration. This is because negative intrathoracic pressure during inspiration leads to increased venous return to the right heart from the IVC and SVC. Ask the patient to sniff if the IVC collapse is not readily apparent, as this may elicit the response. The collapsibility index is a measure of IVC diameter and its percentage decrease during inspiration `Table 8.1`.

M-mode

Measurement of IVC diameter on M-mode echocardiography at end-expiration and end diastole is optional.

Color flow Doppler exam

Examine the hepatic vein (Hv) and the IVC using color flow Doppler
Figures 8.8, 8.9b .

Spectral Doppler exam

Align the PW Doppler sample with the larger hepatic veins that provide an optimal Doppler angle, i.e., the most parallel alignment to the transducer beam
Figure 8.9b .

FINDINGS AND SUMMARIES

See Tables 8.1, 8.3 .

Figure 8.9b

Subcostal views: Color flow Doppler examination of one hepatic vein (Hv, *top*) and the inferior vena cava (IVC, *middle panel*). Note blue flow velocities away from the transducer and toward the right atrium (RA). PW Doppler velocity profiles of both the Hv and IVC show biphasic flow patterns below the baseline. Peak flow velocities mea-sured less than 1 m/s.

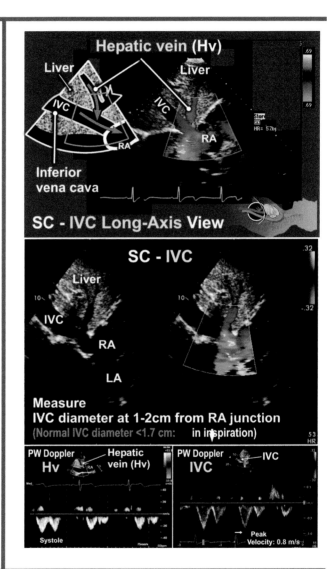

SC-INFERIOR VENA CAVA AND RIGHT ATRIAL PRESSURE ESTIMATES

Table 8.1 ESTIMATION OF RIGHT ATRIAL PRESSURES (RAP) BY ECHOCARDIOGRAPHY

	IVC COLLAPSIBILITY INDEX		
	IVC diameter (cm) *Measure 1–2 cm from RA-IVC junction*	IVC respirophasic movements (inspiratory collapse)	Corresponding RA pressures (mmHg)
Normal	<1.7	≥ 50% or complete inspiratory collapse	5–10
Mild ↑RAP	>1.7 (mildly dilated IVC)	≥ 50% collapse	6–10
Moderate ↑RAP	>1.7 (dilated IVC)	<50% collapse	10–15
Severe ↑RAP	>>1.75 (dilated IVC + hepatic veins)	No collapse	>20
Intravascular volume depletion	<1.2	Spontaneous collapse	<<5

SUBCOSTAL ABDOMINAL AORTA LONG-AXIS (SC-AA-LAX) VIEW

Examination of the abdominal aorta (AA) is a useful adjunct to the subcostal examination. Measurement of the abdominal aortic dimensions is a rapid screening method for detecting aneurysms. Doppler examination of the abdominal aortic flow can provide useful diagnostic information of aortic pathology, including a marker of severity of aortic regurgitation (Figure 6.28).

Patient and transducer positioning

Patient's position remains the same as for the rest of the subcostal examination— with the patient supine and the knees flexed (Figures 8.1, 8.2).

Transducer maneuvers and scan plane orientation

To examine the subcostal long axis of the AA from the SC-IVC-LAX view, maintain the same sagittal scan plane (Figure 8.8). The index mark should be at ~ the 12 o'clock position. Avoid confusing the IVC for the aorta. The abdominal aorta has a hyperechoic (thicker wall) and exhibits visible pulsations. Interrogation with color flow Doppler and PW Doppler can further distinguish both (Figures 8.1, 8.2).

2D scan sector image display

To examine the subcostal long axis of the abdominal aorta (SC-AA-LAX) when starting from the SC-IVC-LAX position, angulate the scan plane toward the left until structures shown in (Figures 8.8 and 8.10) are identified. Identify, optimize, and record the abdominal aorta. The initial branches of the abdominal aorta—the celiac trunk and the superior mesenteric artery—are often visualized.

Color flow Doppler exam

Examine the abdominal aorta using color flow Doppler (Figures 8.8, 8.10).

Spectral Doppler exam

Position the PW Doppler sample within the abdominal aorta at a site that delivers an optimal Doppler angle. Optimize and record abdominal aortic flow. This does not normally exceed 1.35 m/s (Figure 8.10).

Findings and Summaries

See (Table 8.3). Compare dimensions with (Figure 6.27).

SC-ABDOMINAL AORTA LONG AXIS: DOPPLER EXAMINATION
Figure 8.10

Subcostal views: Doppler examination of the abdominal aorta. *Top.* Color flow Doppler examination of the abdominal aorta shows laminar red flow velocities toward the transducer. *Bottom.* PW Doppler examination of the aortic valve shows the characteristic biphasic velocity profiles—with forward flow above the baseline with peak velocities normally below 1.5 m/s.

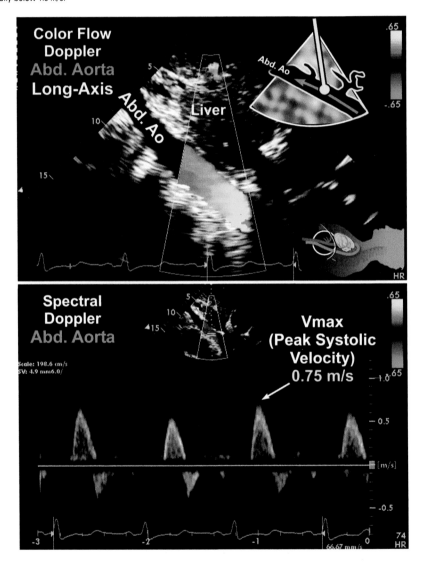

THE SEGMENTAL APPROACH IN PEDIATRIC
ECHOCARDIOGRAPHY AND CONGENITAL HEART DISEASE
Figure 8.11

Congenital heart disease is a complex and highly specialized field. To simplify and standardize the complicated embryological descriptions of the past, a logical sequential segmental analytical approach is now used. Using the sequential segmental analysis method, the sequence of blood flow through the three main cardiac segments are:

1. Atria
2. Ventricles
3. Great arteries

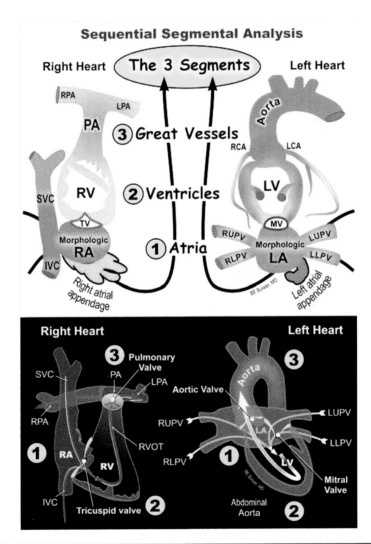

In pediatric cardiology/echocardiography, the normal segments are designated by three letters {S, D, S} that describe the normal arrangement.

- **S:** Situs solitus—signifies a normal atrial and abdominal organ (liver, stomach, spleen) arrangement (site or location) Figure 8.11 . In echocardiography, the subcostal window is used to establish situs. This is the rationale for choice of the subcostal (subxiphoid) window as the starting point in pediatric echocardiography Table 8.2 .
- **D:** D-looping—signifies the normal D-loop (dextro or rightward folding of the embryonic heart tube). This establishes atrioventricular (a-v) concordance—whether the atria and ventricles are attached normally (D-loop) or switched (L-loop). Echocardiographically, the morphologic criteria are used to assign cardiac segments and connections Figure 7.10 ; Table 8.2 .
- **S:** Normal aorto-pulmonary relationship between the great arteries—the main pulmonary artery and the aorta. Echocardiographically, this is established using the PSAX-AVL view Figures 6.40–6.47 .

MORPHOLOGIC CRITERIA IN ASSIGNING SEGMENTS AND CONNECTIONS

Table 8.2 ECHOCARDIOGRAPHIC FEATURES OF CARDIAC SEGMENTS AND CONNECTIONS

Morphologic Right Atrium	Morphologic Left Atrium
• Receives right-sided IVC and SVC • Morphologic right atrial appendage (triangular, broad-based, with pectinate muscles extending outside appendage lumen)	• Receives four (4) pulmonic veins • Attached to left atrial appendage—smaller tubular with pectinate muscles confined to appendage lumen
Tricuspid Valve	**Mitral Valve**
• Trileaflet • Septal leaflet (attached to ventricular septum) • Septal insertion more apical than mitral valve	• Bileaflet • No septal leaflet
Morphologic Right Ventricle	**Morphologic Left Ventricle**
• Coarse trabeculations • Moderator (septomarginal) band • Trileaflet (tricuspid) valve • "Triangular" ventricular cavity • Septal chordae • Infundibular muscle band	• Less coarse trabeculations • Two clearly defined papillary muscles • Ellipsoid ventricular cavity • Bileaflet (mitral) valve
Morphologic Main Pulmonary Artery	**Morphologic Aorta**
• Branch pattern: main trunk with right and left branches	• Coronary arteries (with coronary sinuses) • Aortic arch with arteries to head and neck

SC-4C, INFERIOR VENA CAVA, AND ABDOMINAL AORTA SURVEY: NORMAL AND ABNORMAL FINDINGS

Table 8.3 SUBCOSTAL (SC) VIEWS: THE EXAMINATION SUMMARY

Sequential survey	Findings: subcostal 4-chamber, IVC, and abdominal aorta views (can be used to obtain views equivalent to chest wall windows when such windows are unavailable, as in patients with hyperinflated lung disease [emphysema]; post-major chest wall trauma or surgery)	
	Structural: on 2D, 3D, or M-mode	**Functional and hemodynamic/Doppler**
Left atrium (LA)	• Corroborate findings with the PLAX, A4C, and other views; see Tables 6.1, 7.2 • LA views and measures: Fig. 6.30 , Table 12.6	
Right atrium (RA)	Corroborate findings with the RV inflow view; see Table 6.2 ; Fig. 6.44 • RA enlargement (dilatation) • R atrial masses—most commonly thrombi • Chiari network (embryonic remnant of the sinus venosum— nonpathologic) • Cardiac hardware, e.g., pacemaker/ defibrillator wire—traverses tricuspid valve	Corroborate findings with the RV inflow view; see Table 6.2 • Tricuspid regurgitation (TR) jet on color flow Doppler • Elevated right atrial pressures (RAP) Figs. 4.5, 6.42 ; Table 8.1 **Signs of elevated RAP:** • Dilated IVC with decreased respirophasic collapse—use subcostal-IVC view (see Fig. 8.10 ; Table 8.1) • Dilated tributary veins: IVC, SVC, coronary sinus • Dilated RA, RV • Severe TR • Bowing of interatrial septum to- ward the left (throughout cardiac cycle)
Interatrial septum (IAS)	2D assessment of the interatrial septum Figs. 8.4, 8.8, 8.9 for: • PFO, ASD • Lipomatous hypertrophy of the interatrial septum	• Color flow Doppler to IAS Fig. 8.9 • CW Doppler assessment of flow across IAS • Calculation of shunt size and Qp:Qs (pulmonary-to-systemic flow) ratio
Left ventricle (LV)	• Corroborate findings with the PLAX, PSAX, A4C, and other views: See Table 7.2 • Measures of LV structure and function: Figs. 6.18–6.23 ; Tables 12.1–12.3	

Table 8.3 SUBCOSTAL (SC) VIEWS: THE EXAMINATION SUMMARY *(continued)*

Sequential survey	Findings: subcostal 4-chamber, IVC, and abdominal aorta views (can be used to obtain views equivalent to chest wall windows when such windows are unavailable, as in patients with hyperinflated lung disease [emphysema]; post-major chest wall trauma or surgery)	
	Structural: on 2D, 3D, or M-mode	**Functional and hemodynamic/Doppler**
Right ventricle (RV)	• Corroborate findings with the PLAX, RV inflow, A4C, and other views; see ⬚ Tables 6.1, 7.2 ⬚; RV views ⬚ Figs. 6.31, 6.32 ⬚ • Good view for visualization of the RV free wall • Good for observing myocardial fat pad • Entire long axis of the RVOT can be visualized	
Pericardium	• Pericardial effusion ⬚ Fig. 6.33 ⬚ • Pericardial thickening	• ± tamponade physiology ⬚ Fig. 6.33 ⬚ • ± constrictive physiology
Inferior vena cava (IVC) and intrahepatic veins	• IVC dimensions (see ⬚ Table 8.1 ⬚) • Thrombi	• Respirophasic estimation of right atrial pressures (RAP). Add to pulmonary artery systolic pressure (PASP) measurement derived from applying Bernoulli equation to the CW Doppler-derived peak velocities of the tricuspid regurgitant (TR) jet. (see ⬚ Table 8.1 ⬚; ⬚ Figs. 4.5, 6.2, 6.43a ⬚)
Abdominal aorta	• Aortic dimensions • Aneurysm • Dissection flap	• Diastolic flow reversal (severe AR) by PW to descending thoracic or abdominal aorta ⬚ Figs. 6.27, 6.28 ⬚ • Color flow Doppler: Differential color flow velocities DTAo—in the true and false lumen may be evident in aortic dissection (AD)

CHAPTER 9

Suprasternal Notch (SSN) View

In the comprehensive adult examination, the suprasternal notch (SSN) view facilitates examination of the aortic arch and branches, as well as the descending thoracic aorta [Figures 9.1–9.5]. In the adult examination, the suprasternal notch long-axis (SSN-LAX) view of the aortic arch is mainly used to assess for aortic coarctation, but other parameters of aortic function, e.g., flow reversal in severe aortic regurgitation, should be assessed where indicated [Figures 9.3–9.7].

In pediatric echocardiography, where there is less bony impediment to ultrasound imaging, other views, e.g., aortic arch short-axis views, are routinely sought [Figures 9.8–9.11].

PATIENT AND TRANSDUCER POSITIONING

The patient assumes the supine position with the neck extended, with a pillow placed under the shoulders to promote neck hyperextension. Take care to avoid excessive contraction of the sternocleidomastoid muscle, which can impair transducer positioning. Asking the patient to move the chin to the left or right gives more room for transducer maneuvers. Position the transducer, with acoustic gel, gently but firmly in the suprasternal notch with the transducer index mark directed as shown [Figures 9.1–9.4].

Transducer maneuvers

For the SSN-LAX view of the aortic arch, point the transducer downward in the direction of the long axis of the thoracic aorta, with the index mark pointing toward 1 o'clock [Figures 9.3–9.4].

2D scan sector image display

Identify the ascending aorta, aortic arch and branches, and initial segment of the descending thoracic aorta. Note also the right pulmonary artery as it arches under the aortic arch on its way to the right lung [Figures 9.3–9.5]. Optimize and record the structures of interest [Figure 9.5].

Color flow Doppler exam

Apply color flow Doppler sequentially to the ascending and the descending thoracic aorta Figure 9.6 . Note the normal color flow Doppler patterns. Look for areas of accelerated flow that may indicate aortic stenosis (in the ascending aorta) or coarctation (in the proximal descending thoracic aorta).

The suprasternal notch (SSN) view is the optimal site for spectral Doppler examination of the proximal descending thoracic aorta for suspected coarctation.

Using color flow Doppler as a guide Figure 9.6 , place the PW Doppler sample volume in the proximal descending thoracic aorta to assess proximal flow velocities Figure 9.7 . If flow acceleration (turbulent flow) is seen on color flow Doppler, interrogate proximal and distal to this region to detect any increase in blood flow velocities. Use continuous-wave (CW) Doppler to detect peak flow velocities across this region Figure 9.7 .

Findings and Summaries

Assess cardiac structure and function. Confirm findings on complementary views Table 7.2 .

SSN-AORTIC ARCH LONG-AXIS VIEW: PATIENT POSITIONING AND TRANSDUCER PLACEMENT

Figure 9.1

Patient and transducer positioning: suprasternal notch (SSN) window.

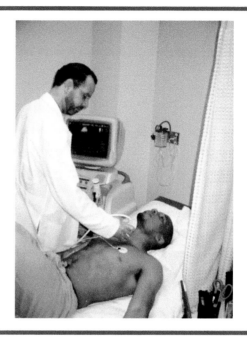

Figure 9.2

Patient and transducer positioning. Suprasternal notch (SSN) window. Note the transducer index mark pointing to approximately the 1 o'clock position.

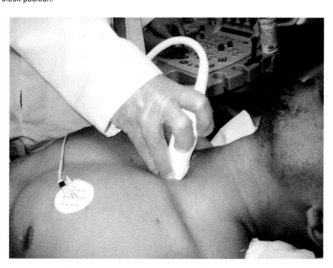

SSN AORTIC ARCH LONG-AXIS SCAN PLANE ANATOMY

Figure 9.3

Suprasternal long-axis scan planes anatomical view (left) and lateral view (right).

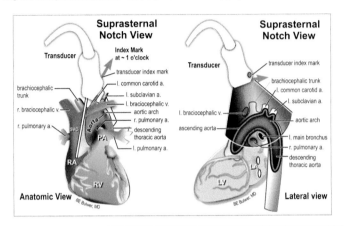

Figure 9.4

Suprasternal notch (SSN) long-axis scan plane: posterior perspective.

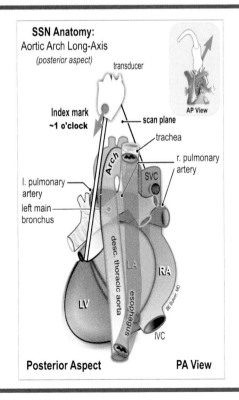

SSN AORTIC ARCH LONG-AXIS SCAN SECTOR ANATOMY
Figure 9.5

Suprasternal notch long-axis view. Note the dense echoreflectivity of the air-filled left main bronchus below the aortic arch.

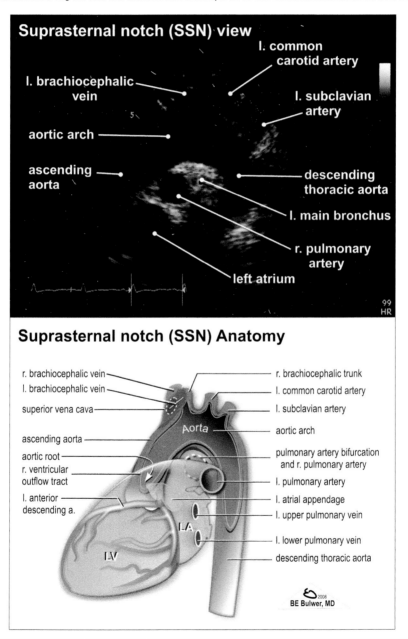

Suprasternal notch (SSN) view

I. common carotid artery

I. brachiocephalic vein

I. subclavian artery

aortic arch

ascending aorta

descending thoracic aorta

I. main bronchus

r. pulmonary artery

left atrium

99
HR

Suprasternal notch (SSN) Anatomy

r. brachiocephalic vein
I. brachiocephalic vein
superior vena cava
ascending aorta
aortic root
r. ventricular outflow tract
I. anterior descending a.

Aorta

LA

LV

r. brachiocephalic trunk
I. common carotid artery
I. subclavian artery
aortic arch
pulmonary artery bifurcation and r. pulmonary artery
I. pulmonary artery
I. atrial appendage
I. upper pulmonary vein
I. lower pulmonary vein
descending thoracic aorta

2008
BE Bulwer, MD

SSN AORTIC ARCH LONG AXIS: COLOR DOPPLER EXAMINATION

Figure 9.6

Suprasternal notch (SSN) long axis. Color flow Doppler examination. Compare with Figure 4.9.

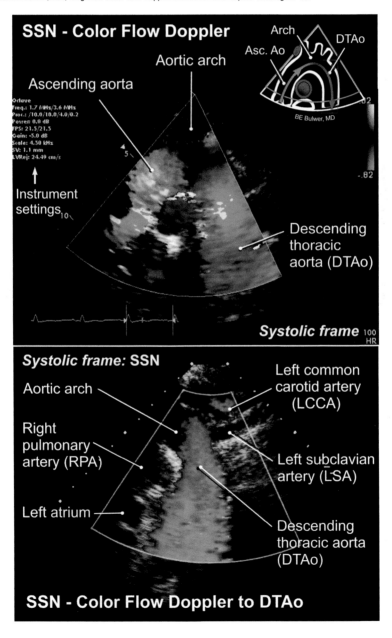

SSN AORTIC ARCH LONG-AXIS: SPECTRAL DOPPLER EXAMINATION
Figure 9.7

Suprasternal notch (SSN) long-axis view: *(top)* pulsed-wave (PW) Doppler and *(bottom)* continuous-wave Doppler interrogation of the descending thoracic aorta (DTAo).

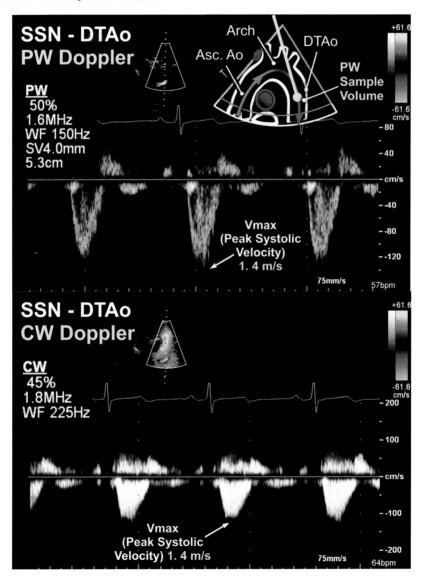

SSN AORTIC ARCH LONG-AXIS SURVEY: NORMAL AND ABNORMAL FINDINGS

Table 9.1 SUPRASTERNAL NOTCH (SSN) VIEWS: THE EXAMINATION SUMMARY

Sequential survey	*Findings:* <u>Suprasternal notch views</u>	
	Structural: on 2D, 3D, or M-Mode	**Functional and hemodynamic**
Aorta	LONG AXIS: ASCENDING AORTA AND ARCH `Fig. 6.27` • Dimensions: dilatation—aneurysm • Dissection: flap • Atheroma/calcification AORTIC ARCH AND GREAT ARTERIES *(Brachiocephalic trunk [usually outside imaging plane]; left common carotid, left subclavian artery–LSA)* • Aneurysm • Dissection • Atheroma • Coarctation (distal to LSA) DESCENDING THORACIC AORTA • Coarctation of the aorta SHORT AXIS `Figs. 9.8–9.11` • SVC, aortic arch, right PA immediately posterior and inferior to the ascending aorta/aortic arch	• Doppler assessment; color, PW and CW as appropriate `Figs. 6.28, 6.29` • Diastolic flow reversal (severe AR) `Fig. 6.28` • Flow acceleration seen on color flow Doppler; increased gradient
LA	• Sometimes visualized below the RPA	• Generally not assessed on SSN view
Right pulmonary artery	• Occasional thrombus or saddle embolus • Catheter (Swan-Ganz)	Estimation of right-sided pressures `Figs. 4.5, 6.42`

SSN AORTIC ARCH SHORT-AXIS SCAN PLANE ANATOMY
Figure 9.8

Suprasternal notch short-axis window: transducer position and scan planes.

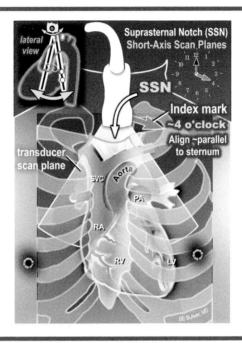

Figure 9.9

Suprasternal notch short-axis scan planes: *(left)* ascending aortic frontal plane and *(right)* aortic arch short-axis and "crab" view.

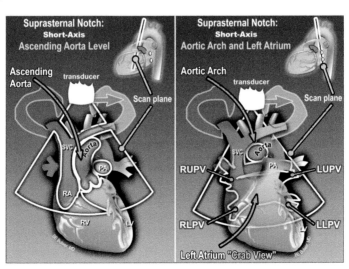

SSN AORTIC ARCH SHORT AXIS: ASCENDING AORTIC FRONTAL VIEW
Figure 9.10

Suprasternal notch short-axis view: ascending aortic frontal plane.

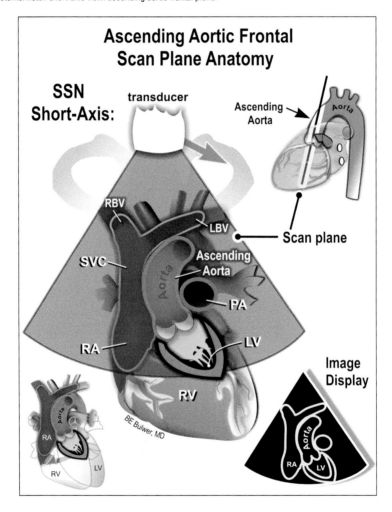

SSN AORTIC ARCH SHORT AXIS: "CRAB" VIEW
Figure 9.11

Suprasternal notch short-axis view: aortic arch short-axis and "crab" view.

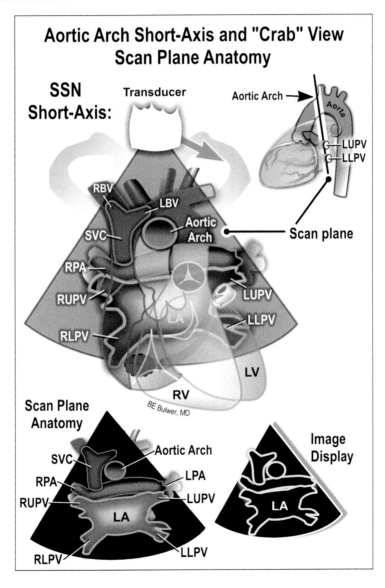

CHAPTER 10

Right Parasternal Long-Axis View (R-PLAX)

INTRODUCTION

In the adult transthoracic examination, the right parasternal long-axis (R-PLAX) window is an alternative site for optimal assessment of the severity of aortic stenosis Figures 2.4, 6.29 . On this view, a parallel alignment of the ascending aorta, the aortic valve (AV), and the initial portion of the left ventricular outflow tract (LVOT) can be achieved Figure 10.1 . This alignment facilitates optimal assessment of peak flow velocities across the aortic valve in patients with aortic stenosis, especially when other views are inadequate, or there is reason to suspect that was underestimation of peak trans-aortic flow velocities on previous views Figures 6.29, 10.2 .

In the pediatric examination, the high R-PLAX view can be used to assess the right atrium and its tributaries—the superior (SVC) and inferior vena cavae (IVC), as well as the interatrial septum (IAS) Figure 10.1 . From this window, the IAS separating the RA and the LA is generally well aligned for visualization of atrial septal defects Figure 6.44 . The right pulmonary artery as it passes behind the superior vena cava Figure 10.1 , and the right upper pulmonary vein, can also be seen.

Figure 10.1

The right parasternal long-axis view. *Above left.* High right parasternal long-axis scan plane. *Above right.* Right parasternal long-axis perspective showing the optimal Doppler alignment of the ascending aorta, the aortic valve, and the left ventricular outflow tract (LVOT). *Below left.* Posteriorly directed scan plane from the right parasternal window. This view is useful for visualization and assessment of the structures depicted in the neonatal and pediatric examination. *Below right.* Note corresponding scan plane anatomy and corresponding scan sector display outline. *IVC: inferior vena cava; LA: left atrium; RA: right atrium; LVOT: left ventricular outflow tract; RPA: right pulmonary artery; RUPV: right upper pulmonary vein.*

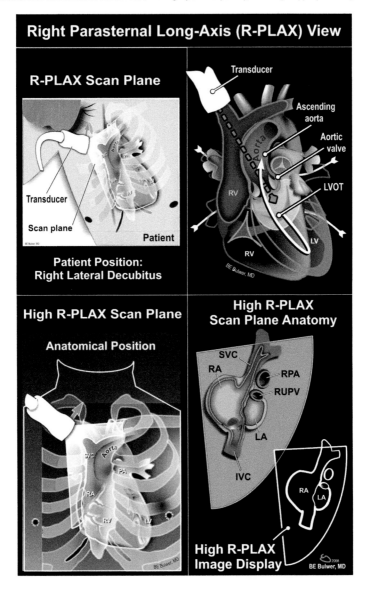

PATIENT AND TRANSDUCER POSITIONING

The right parasternal view may be the most difficult to obtain. There is no cardiac notch (lung free space near the right sterna border (see Figures 2.4, 2.11, 2.12). Therefore the presence of the air filled lung, as well as the bony sternum, can make imaging technically difficult. Following assessment of aortic stenosis using the standard views Figure 6.29 , position patient in the right lateral decubitus position with the patient lying comfortably and the right hand folded under the head, akin the left lateral decubitus position Figures 2.11, 2.12, 6.6a, 10.1 .

Position the transducer anywhere from the 2nd to the 4th right intercostal space. Direct the transducer beam under the sternum and toward the cardiac apex. This should approximate a line parallel to the ascending aorta and directed toward the left ventricular (LV) apex Figure 10.1 . Initially, use the standard full-modality imaging transducer followed by color flow Doppler to the region of interest. Then assess peak flow velocities by continuous-wave (CW) Doppler using a dedicated non-imaging (pencil) probe or Pedoff transducer.

Transducer maneuvers

When using a standard imaging probe, initial identification of the ascending aorta and color flow Doppler should be used as a guide. When a dedicated non-imaging transducer is used, maneuver probe and fine-tune until a clear spectral Doppler trace is seen Figure 10.2 or until an optimal ("crisp") Doppler audio signal is heard.

2D scan sector image display

Identify the ascending aorta Figure 10.2 . The cross section at this site should ideally include the proximal ascending aorta, the aortic valve, and that portion of the LVOT immediately. Optimize and record the structures of interest.

Color flow Doppler exam

Apply color flow Doppler to the ascending thoracic aorta Figure 10.2 . With significant aortic stenosis, flow acceleration or turbulent, mosaic flow can be seen on color flow Doppler Figures 6.29, 10.2 .

Spectral Doppler exam

The right parasternal long-axis view can be the optimal view for spectral Doppler examination of peak trans-aortic velocities in patients with aortic stenosis Figure 10.2 . Using first the full-modality imaging probe followed by the dedicated non-imaging probe—search for the highest peak velocities across the aortic valve.

Parallel alignment of the ultrasound beam and the region of interest will optimize the detection of the maximum measurable velocities. Therefore use color flow Doppler as a guide Figure 10.2 , and then place the CW Doppler sample volume across the aortic valve, ensuring optimal parallel alignment of the LVOT. Assess the peak flow velocities across the aortic valve using continuous-wave (CW) Doppler Figure 10.2 .

R-PLAX: SCAN PLANE, ANATOMY, AND DOPPLER EVALUATION
Figure 10.2

Examination of the aortic valve in a patient with aortic stenosis from the right parasternal long-axis view (R-PLAX). Its major advantage is its optimal alignment when evaluating aortic valve (AV) hemodynamics. In this regard, it can more accurately assess aortic stenotic lesions. *Above left.* Optimal Doppler beam alignment with the aortic valve and LVOT. *Above right.* R-PLAX view showing thickened aortic valve in a patient with aortic stenosis. *Middle left.* Color flow Doppler systolic frame of patient with aortic stenosis showing high-flow systolic jet because of aortic stenosis. *Middle right.* Continuous-wave Doppler interrogation of the aortic stenosis jet revealed peak transaortic velocity measuring 5–3 m/s, corresponding to a transaortic pressure gradient exceeding 110 mmHg—consistent with severe aortic stenosis. *Below left.* By contrast, note the appearance of the same jet on the apical 5-chamber (A5C) view. *Below right.* By contrast, note the peak velocity measuring only 3.2 m/s on the A5C view—a severe underestimate.

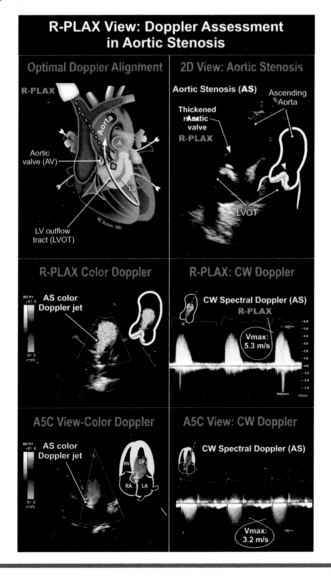

CHAPTER 11

Echocardiography in the Age of Ultra-Portability

THE "ULTRASOUND STETHOSCOPE"

A new dawn has emerged in echocardiography with the advent of highly portable laptop-sized instruments called hand-carried ultrasound (HCU) Figure 1.1 . Further miniaturization into ultra-portable pocket-sized versions Figure 11.1 has given new meaning to the word stetho*scope*—the ability to sonographically see (and not simply listen to) the heart.

Such ultra-portability presents a new paradigm in medical and allied health education, with the prospect of rapidly assessing basic cardiac structure and function at a patient's bedside or at the point-of-care.

This evolution in technology, coupled with new applications in the emergency, community, and far flung settings in today's communication age—presents the prospect of a new era of the "smartphone" of cardiac imaging.

Instrument Features

Current devices generally have simpler instrument controls and are battery powered, with the prime advantages being reduced costs and ultra-portability. B-mode (anatomical) imaging is the standard basic feature of such systems, but the addition of color flow Doppler imaging should be the minimum requirement for a truly useful echocardiographic instrument. Spectral (pulsed and continuous-wave) Doppler, tissue Doppler, and 3D features are generally absent, and they have limited ability to store and analyze the acquired data.

Utility versus Competency

The American Society of Echocardiography supports the concept of hand-carried ultrasound systems primarily as an extension of the physical examination, and it recommends at least Level 1 training in echocardiography to ensure competency and safe use of this increasingly available technology Table 11.1 .

Figure 11.1

Hand-carried and pocket-sized hand-held echocardiography instruments. The models shown are manufactured by General Electric, Sonosite, Siemens, and Signostics. Other exciting models are in the pipeline.

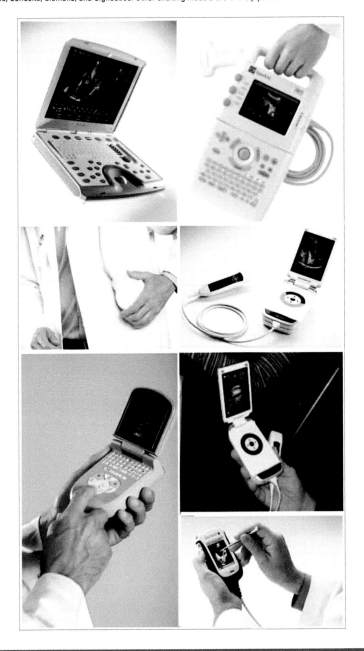

UTILITY AND PERSONNEL

Caution is necessary with the introduction of any new technology into medical training and healthcare. However, a wide array of non-cardiologists are making more use of this increasingly available technology. They range from medical students to doctors at all levels of training, and over an increasing spectrum of specialties, especially in emergency medicine, intensive and critical care. As echocardiography is a sonographic exposé of cardiac structure and function, it is conceptually an ideal tool to use to complement both our understanding of in vivo cardiac anatomy as well as an extension of the bedside physical examination (Figure 11.2).

Figure 11.2

The promise of point-of-care echocardiography: a tool for teaching cardiovascular anatomy and as an adjunct to the bedside cardiac examination.

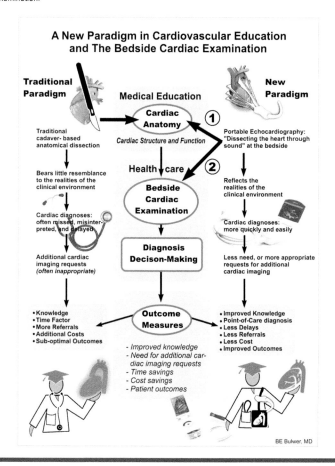

A New Paradigm in Cardiovascular Education and The Bedside Cardiac Examination

BE Bulwer, MD

LEVELS OF TRAINING IN ECHOCARDIOGRAPHY

Table 11.1

	Objectives	Duration	No. of cases
Physicians in cardiology training programs			
Level 1	Introductory experience	3 months	150 2D/M-mode examinations 75 Doppler examinations
Level 2	Sufficient experience to take responsibility for echocardiographic studies	3 additional months (beyond Level 1)	150 2D/M-mode examinations; 150 Doppler examinations
Level 3	Sufficient expertise to direct an echocardiography laboratory	6 additional months (beyond Level 2)	450 examinations (using both imaging and Doppler)
Physicians in post-cardiology training			
	Responsibility for performance and interpretation of echocardiograms	Variable; level of achievement equivalent to Level 2 above	250-300 patients (2D/M-mode and Doppler examinations)
	Direct echo laboratory in practice hospital or large group	Variable; Level of expertise equivalent to level 3	Doppler examinations 450 patients (2D/ M-mode and Doppler

Reference Guide

PART 3

Reference Guide

THE ECHOCARDIOGRAPHY EXAMINATION REPORT
Figure 12.1

Sample transthoracic echocardiography examination report.

The Hospital
Echocardiography Laboratory

Name: Hope Flowers	Sex: M	Study Date: 1/24/2008
MRN #: 01000101	DOB: 2/20/1945	Study Time: 3:29:33 PM
	Age 62 years	Report Date: 1/24/2008
Tech/Fellow: bebjr	Ht: 65.00	Report 4:59:25 PM

Tape #: 12345
Wt: 177.00   BP: 118 / 76 mmHg
BSA: 1.88 kg/m²

Ref. Physician: Dr. Ineed Helpquick
Indications: Evaluation of Structure and Function: LV Function Evaluation
Study Details: Complete Echo (2D, Color Flow, Doppler) - 993303. Outpatient.

Diagnosis: CHF 421.0; CP

2D MEASUREMENTS:
IVS, d	0.20 cm		
LVID, d	5.20 cm	LV Mass (AL)	173.5 g
LVID, s	3.70 cm	LV Mass (BSA)	92.4 g/m²
LVPW, d	0.90 cm	Aortic Root, d	3.70 cm
LA, s	4.60 cm		

Left Ventricle: The left ventricle is normal in size. There is borderline concentric left ventricular hypertrophy with basal posterior thinning. Overall left ventricular function is normal. The estimated ejection fraction is 65%. Ejection fraction by bi-plane method (Simpson's) = 67% .

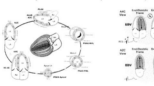

Right Ventricle: Normal right ventricular size, wall thickness, and contractility.
Left Atrium: There is mild left atrial enlargement. The interatrial septum normal.
Right Atrium: Normal right atrial size.

Aortic Valve: The aortic valve is structurally normal and trileaflet. There is no aortic insufficiency with a posteriorly-directed jet.
Mitral Valve: The mitral valve is mildly diffusely thickened. There is trace mitral regurgitation.

Tricuspid Valve: The tricuspid valve is structurally normal. There is trace tricuspid regurgitation. The tricuspid regurgitant velocity is 2.53 m/s, consistent with a normal pulmonary artery systolic pressure of 25 mmHg plus right atrial pressure.

Pulmonic Valve: Structurally normal pulmonic valve. There is trace pulmonic regurgitation.

Aorta: The aortic root size is normal.

Pulmonary Artery: The main pulmonary artery appears normal in size.

Venous: The inferior vena cava diameter is normal; normal inspiratory collapse

Pericardium/Pleura: There is no significant pericardial effusion.
Prior studies: A prior study was performed on 03/22/02. Compared with the prior report, there has been no significant change.

Supervising/Interpreting Physician: Johnny B. Goode MD, PhD

Johnny B. Goode MD, PhD

ECHOCARDIOGRAPHIC CORRELATES OF NORMAL INTRACARDIAC PRESSURES

Figure 12.2

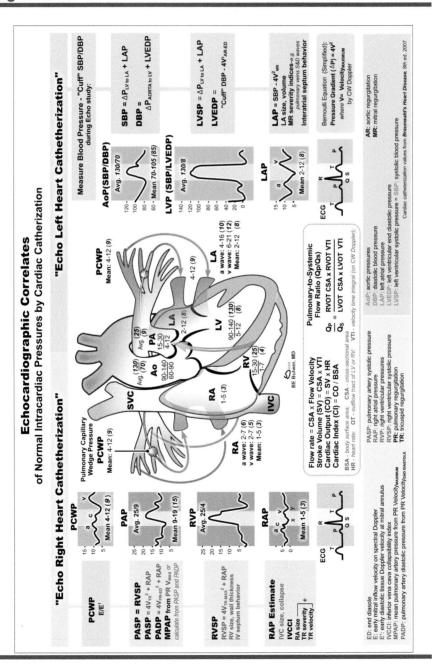

Echocardiographic Correlates of Normal Intracardiac Pressures by Cardiac Catheterization

Table 12.1 REFERENCE LIMITS AND PARTITION VALUES
OF LEFT VENTRICULAR (LV) SIZE

	Women				Men			
	Reference range	Mildly abnormal	Moderately abnormal	Severely abnormal	Reference range	Mildly abnormal	Moderately abnormal	Severely abnormal
LV Dimension								
LV diastolic diameter	3.9-5.3	5.4-5.7	5.8-6.1	≥ 6.2	4.2-5.9	6.0-6.3	6.4-6.8	≥ 6.9
LV diastolic diameter/ BSA (cm/m^2)	2.4-3.2	3.3-3.4	3.5-3.7	≥ 3.8	2.2-3.1	3.2-3.4	3.5-3.6	≥ 3.7
LV diastolic diameter/ height (cm/m)	2.5-3.2	3.3-3.4	3.5-3.6	≥ 3.7	2.4-3.3	3.4-3.5	3.6-3.7	≥ 3.8
LV Volume								
LV diastolic volume (ml)	56-104	105-117	118-180	> 131	67-155	156-178	179-200	> 201
LV diastolic volume/ BSA (ml/m^2)	*35-75*	*76-86*	*87-96*	*≥ 97*	*35-75*	*76-86*	*87-96*	*≥ 97*
LV systolic volume (ml)	19-49	50-59	60-69	≥ 70	22-58	59-70	71-82	≥ 83
LV systolic volume/ BSA (ml/m^2)	*12-30*	*31-36*	*37-42*	*≥ 43*	*12-30*	*31-36*	*37-42*	*≥ 43*
Highlighted values: Recommended and best validated								

Table 12.2 REFERENCE LIMITS AND PARTITION VALUES
OF LEFT VENTRICULAR (LV) FUNCTION

	Women				Men			
	Reference range	Mildly abnormal	Moderately abnormal	Severely abnormal	Reference range	Mildly abnormal	Moderately abnormal	Severely abnormal
Linear Method								
Endocardial fractional shortening (%)	27-45	22-26	17-21	≤ 16	25-43	20-24	15-19	≤ 14
Midwall fractional shortening (%)	15-23	13-14	11-12	≤ 10	14-22	12-13	10-11	≤ 10
2D Method								
Ejection fraction (%)	*≥ 55*	*45-54*	*30-44*	*< 30*	*≥ 55*	*45-54*	*30-44*	*< 30*
Highlighted values: Recommended and best validated								

LEFT VENTRICULAR MASS AND GEOMETRY

Table 12.3 REFERENCE LIMITS AND PARTITION VALUES OF LEFT VENTRICULAR MASS AND GEOMETRY

	Women				Men			
	Reference Range	Mildly Abnormal	Moderately Abnormal	Severely Abnormal	Reference Range	Mildly Abnormal	Moderately Abnormal	Severely Abnormal
Linear Methods								
LV mass (g)	67-162	163-186	187-210	≥211	88-224	225-258	259-292	≥293
LV mass/BSA (g/m²)	*43-95*	*96-108*	*109-121*	*≥122*	*49-115*	*116-131*	*132-148*	*≥149*
LV mass/height (g/m)	41-99	100-115	116-128	≥129	52-126	127-144	145-162	≥163
LV mass/height$^{2.7}$ (g/m)$^{2.7}$	18-44	45-51	52-58	≥59	20-48	49-55	56-63	≥64
Relative wall thickness (cm)	0.22-0.42	0.43-0.47	0.48-0.52	≥0.53	0.24-0.42	0.43-0.46	0.47-0.51	≥0.52
Septal thickness (cm)	*0.6-0.9*	*1.0-1.2*	*1.3-1.5*	*≥1.6*	*0.6-1.0*	*1.1-1.3*	*1.4-1.6*	*≥1.7*
Posterior Wall Thickness (cm)	*0.6-0.9*	*1.0-1.2*	*1.3-1.5*	*≥1.6*	*0.6-1.0*	*1.1-1.3*	*1.4-1.6*	*≥1.7*
2D Methods								
LV mass (g)	66-150	151-171	172-182	>193	96-200	201-227	228-254	>255
LV mass/BSA (g/m²)	*44-88*	*89-100*	*101-112*	*≥113*	*50-102*	*103-116*	*117-130*	*≥131*

RIGHT VENTRICULAR SIZE AND FUNCTION

Table 12.4 REFERENCE LIMITS AND PARTITION VALUES OF RIGHT VENTRICULAR SIZE AND FUNCTION AS MEASURED IN THE APICAL FOUR-CHAMBER VIEW.

	Reference Range	Mildly Abnormal	Moderately Abnormal	Severely Abnormal
RV Diastolic Area (cm^2)	11–28	29–32	33–37	≥38
RV Systolic Area (cm^2)	7.5–16	17–19	20–22	≥23
RV Fractional Area Change (%)	32–60	25–31	18–24	≥17

RV, Right ventricular. Weyman A. Practices and principles of echocardiography. 2nd ed. Philadelphia: Lippincott, Williams and Wilkins; 1994.

RIGHT VENTRICULAR AND PULMONARY ARTERY SIZE

Table 12.5 REFERENCE LIMITS AND PARTITION/VALUES OF RIGHT VENTRICULAR (RV) AND PULMONARY ARTERY (PA) SIZE

	Reference range	Mildly abnormal	Moderately abnormal	Severely abnormal
RV DIMENSIONS				
Basal RV diameter (RVD#1) (cm)	2.0–2.8	2.9–3.3	3.4–3.8	≥16
Mid RV diameter (RVD#2) (cm)	2.7–3.3	3.4–3.7	3.8–4.1	≥4.2
Base-to-apex length (RVD#3) (cm)	7.1–7.9	8.0–8.5	8.6–9.1	≥9.2
RVOT DIAMETERS				
Above aortic valve (RVOT#1) (cm)	2.5–2.9	3.0–3.2	3.3–3.5	≥3.6
Above pulmonic valve (RVOT#2) (cm)	1.7–2.3	2.4–2.7	2.8–3.1	≥3.2
PA DIAMETER				
Below pulmonic valve (PA#1) (cm)	1.5–2.1	2.2–2.5	2.6–2.9	≥3.0

RV, Right ventricular; *RVOT,* right ventricular outflow tract; *PA,* pulmonary artery. Foale R, Nihoyannopoulos P, McKenna W, Kleinebenne A, Nadazdin A, Rowland E, et al. Echocardiographic measurement of the normal adult right ventricle. *Br Heart J* 1986;56:33–44.

LEFT ATRIAL DIMENSIONS AND VOLUMES

Table 12.6 REFERENCE LIMITS AND PARTITION VALUES OF LEFT ATRIAL (LA) DIMENSIONS/VOLUMES

	Women				Men			
	Reference range	Mildly abnormal	Moderately abnormal	Severely abnormal	Reference range	Mildly abnormal	Moderately abnormal	Severely abnormal
ATRIAL DIMENSIONS								
LA diameter (cm)	2.7–3.8	3.9–4.2	4.3–4.6	≥4.7	3.0–4.0	4.1–4.6	4.7–5.2	≥5.2
LA diameter/BSA (cm/m^2)	1.5–2.3	2.4–2.6	2.7–2.9	≥3.0	1.5–2.3	2.4–2.6	2.7–2.9	≥3.0
RA minor axis dimension (cm)	2.9–4.5	4.6–4.9	5.0–5.4	≥5.5	2.9–4.5	4.6–4.9	5.0–5.4	≥5.5
RA minor axis dimension/BSA (cm/m^2)	1.7–2.5	2.6–2.8	2.9–3.1	≥3.2	1.7–2.5	2.6–2.8	2.9–3.1	≥3.2
ATRIAL AREA								
LA area (cm^2)	≤20	20–30	30–40	>40	≤20	20–30	30–40	>40
ATRIAL VOLUMES								
LA volume (ml)	22–52	53–62	63–72	≥73	18–58	59–68	69–78	≥79
LA volume/BSA (ml/m^2)	*22±6*	*29–33*	*34–39*	*≥40*	*22±6*	*29–33*	*34–39*	*≥40*

STRESS ECHOCARDIOGRAPHY
Figure 12.3

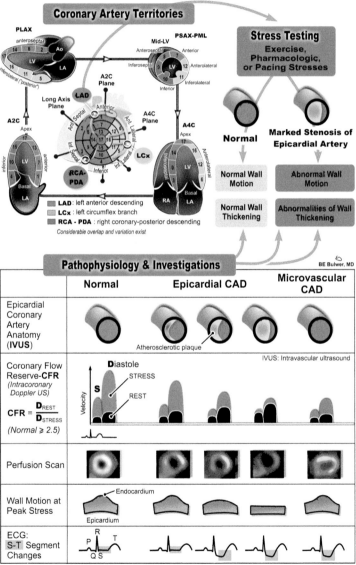

Stress Echocardiography
Coronary Artery Disease (CAD) and Basic Principles of Stress Testing

Coronary Artery Territories

Stress Testing
Exercise, Pharmacologic, or Pacing Stresses

Normal — Marked Stenosis of Epicardial Artery

Normal Wall Motion — Abnormal Wall Motion

Normal Wall Thickening — Abnormalities of Wall Thickening

LAD: left anterior descending
LCx : left circumflex branch
RCA - PDA : right coronary-posterior descending
Considerable overlap and variation exist

BE Bulwer, MD

Pathophysiology & Investigations

	Normal	Epicardial CAD	Microvascular CAD
Epicardial Coronary Artery Anatomy (**IVUS**)		Atherosclerotic plaque	IVUS: Intravascular ultrasound
Coronary Flow Reserve-**CFR** (*Intracoronary Doppler US*) $CFR = \dfrac{D_{REST}}{D_{STRESS}}$ (*Normal* ⩾ 2.5)	Diastole / STRESS / S / REST		
Perfusion Scan			
Wall Motion at Peak Stress	Endocardium / Epicardium		
ECG: **S-T** Segment Changes	R / P / T / Q S		

Standardized Myocardial Segmentation and Nomenclature. *Circulation* 2002;105:539-42   Picano E. *Stress Echocardiography*, 5th ed. Springer, Berlin, 2009: 31-42

Figure 12.4

Stress Echocardiography and Wall Motion Assessment

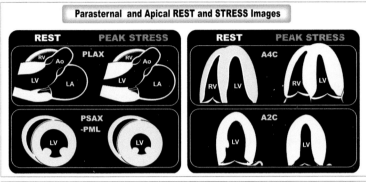

Parasternal and Apical REST and STRESS Images

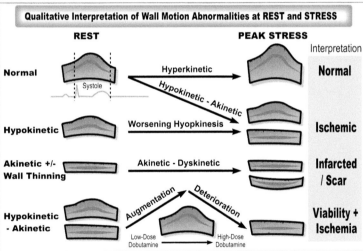

Qualitative Interpretation of Wall Motion Abnormalities at REST and STRESS

BE Bulwer, MD

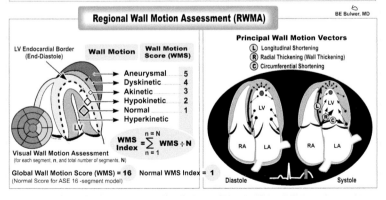

Regional Wall Motion Assessment (RWMA)

Figure 12.5

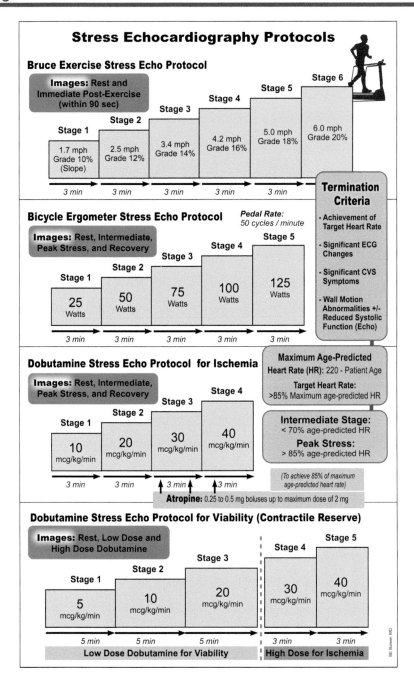

Stress Echocardiography Protocols

Bruce Exercise Stress Echo Protocol

Images: Rest and Immediate Post-Exercise (within 90 sec)

Stage 1: 1.7 mph Grade 10% (Slope)
Stage 2: 2.5 mph Grade 12%
Stage 3: 3.4 mph Grade 14%
Stage 4: 4.2 mph Grade 16%
Stage 5: 5.0 mph Grade 18%
Stage 6: 6.0 mph Grade 20%

3 min | 3 min | 3 min | 3 min | 3 min

Bicycle Ergometer Stress Echo Protocol
Pedal Rate: 50 cycles / minute

Images: Rest, Intermediate, Peak Stress, and Recovery

Stage 1: 25 Watts
Stage 2: 50 Watts
Stage 3: 75 Watts
Stage 4: 100 Watts
Stage 5: 125 Watts

3 min | 3 min | 3 min | 3 min | 3 min

Termination Criteria
- Achievement of Target Heart Rate
- Significant ECG Changes
- Significant CVS Symptoms
- Wall Motion Abnormalities +/- Reduced Systolic Function (Echo)

Dobutamine Stress Echo Protocol for Ischemia

Images: Rest, Intermediate, Peak Stress, and Recovery

Stage 1: 10 mcg/kg/min
Stage 2: 20 mcg/kg/min
Stage 3: 30 mcg/kg/min
Stage 4: 40 mcg/kg/min

3 min | 3 min | 3 min | 3 min

Maximum Age-Predicted Heart Rate (HR): 220 - Patient Age
Target Heart Rate: >85% Maximum age-predicted HR

Intermediate Stage: < 70% age-predicted HR
Peak Stress: > 85% age-predicted HR

(To achieve 85% of maximum age-predicted heart rate)

Atropine: 0.25 to 0.5 mg boluses up to maximum dose of 2 mg

Dobutamine Stress Echo Protocol for Viability (Contractile Reserve)

Images: Rest, Low Dose and High Dose Dobutamine

Stage 1: 5 mcg/kg/min
Stage 2: 10 mcg/kg/min
Stage 3: 20 mcg/kg/min
Stage 4: 30 mcg/kg/min
Stage 5: 40 mcg/kg/min

5 min | 5 min | 5 min | 3 min | 3 min

Low Dose Dobutamine for Viability | **High Dose for Ischemia**

BE Bulwer MD

STRESS ECHOCARDIOGRAPHY

Table 12.7 STRESS ECHOCARDIOGRAPHY: UTILITY AND INDICATIONS

Protocol		Utility	Indications/Comments
Exercise Stress Echocardiography	Treadmill, Bicycle: supine or upright	Diagnostic	Patients with abnormal baseline ECG or limited exercise tolerance • Non-specific ST-T-wave changes • Left bundle branch block • Left ventricular hypertrophy • Digoxin therapy • Wolf-Parkinson-White syndrome
		Prognostic	• Chronic Coronary Artery Disease • Post-myocardial Infarction
		Risk Stratification	• In heart failure: contractile reserve, mitral valve function, right ventricular function • Perioperative evaluation for non-cardiac surgery
Pharmacologic Stress Echocardiography	Sympathomimetic amines e.g. Dobutamine ($\pm$ atropine)— agent of choice (USA)	As for Exercise Stress Echocardiography (in patients unable to exercise)	• Indications as for Exercise Stress Echocardiography (when patients unable to exercise) • Myocardial viability assessment (for biphasic response) • Contractile reserve in patients with heart failure and low-gradient aortic stenosis
	Vasodilators e.g. Dypridamole, Adenosine	As for Exercise Stress Echocardiography (in patients unable to exercise)	Less sensitivity than with sympathomimetic amines (used mainly outside the USA)
	Other; Ergonovine-Ergometrine, Enoximone	Evaluation of vasospastic coronary artery disease	
Pacing Stress Echocardiography	Atrial	Diagnostic option for patients with known or suspected coronary artery disease (some centers)	
	Transesophageal atrial pacing		
Stress Echocardiography with Doppler	Exercise treadmill, Supine bicycle	Low gradient aortic stenosis (with left ventricular dysfunction)	Assessment of contractile reserve (Dobutamine stress)
		Heart failure; Assessment of systolic/diastolic dysfunction	Mitral regurgitation and Transmitral Doppler indices using exercise or pharmacologic protocols

STRESS ECHOCARDIOGRAPHY

Table 12.8 NORMAL AND ISCHEMIC RESPONSES FOR VARIOUS MODALITIES OF STRESS (ASE, 2007)

Stress method	Regional		Global	
	Normal response	Ischemic response	Normal response	Ischemic response
Treadmill	Postexercise increase in function compared with rest	Postexercise decrease in function compared with rest	Decrease in ESV, increase in EF	Increase in ESV, decrease in EF in multivessel or L main disease
Supine bicycle	Peak exercise increase in function compared with rest	Peak exercise decrease in function compared with rest	Decrease in ESV, increase in EF	Increase in ESV and decrease in EF in multivessel or L main disease
Dobutamine	Increase in function, velocity of contraction compared with rest and usually with low dose	Decrease in function, velocity of contraction compared with low dose; may be less compared with rest	Greater decrease in ESV, marked increase in EF	Often same as normal response; infrequently, ischemia produces decreased EF; cavity dilatation rarely occurs
Vasodilator	Increase in function compared with rest	Decrease in function compared with rest	Decrease in ESV, increase in EF	Often same as normal response; occasionally, ischemia produces decreased EF; cavity dilatation rarely occurs
Atrial pacing	No change or increase in function compared with rest	Decrease in function compared with rest	Decrease in ESV, no change in EF	No change or increase in ESV, decrease in EF

EF, Ejection fraction; *ESV,* end-systolic volume; *L,* left.
Reference: Pellikka PA, Nagueh SF, Elhendy AA, Kuehl CA, Sawada SG; American Society of Echocardiography. American Society of Echocardiography recommendations for performance, interpretation, and application of stress echocardiography. *J Am Soc Echocardiogr.* 2007 Sep;20(9): 1021–41.

REFERENCES

Chapter 1: Basic Types of Echocardiography

1. Bulwer BE, Rivero J, Solomon SD. Basic principles of echocardiography and tomographic anatomy. In: Solomon SD (ed.), Braunwald E (series ed). *Atlas of Echocardiography*, 2nd ed. Philadelphia: Current Science; 2008:1–24.

2. Bulwer BE, Shernan SK, Thomas J. Physics of echocardiography. In: Savage RM (ed.), et al. *Comprehensive Textbook of Intraoperative Transesophageal Echocardiography*. Philadelphia: Lippincott Williams & Wilkins; 2010.

Chapter 1: Clinical Value of Echocardiography

1. Douglas PS, Khandheria B, Stainback RF, et al. ACCF/ASE/ACEP/ASNC/ SCAI/SCCT/SCMR 2007 appropriateness criteria for transthoracic and transesophageal echocardiography: a report. *J Am Coll Cardiol.* 2007;50:187–204.

2. Bulwer BE, Shamshad F, Solomon SD. Clinical Utility of Echocardiography. In: Solomon SD (ed.), Bulwer BE (assoc. ed). *Essential Echocardiography. A Practical Casebook with DVD*. Totowa, NJ: Humana Press; 2007:71–86.

Chapter 1: Skills and Competency: The Requisites

1. Ehler D, Carney DK, Dempsey AL, et al. American Society of Echocardiography Sonographer Training and Education Committee. Guidelines for cardiac sonographer education: recommendations of the American Society of Echocardiography Sonographer Training and Education Committee. *J Am Soc Echocardiogr.* 2001;14:77–84.

2. Quiñones MA, Douglas PS, Foster E, et al. ACC; AHA; ACP; ASIM Task Force on Clinical Competence. American College of Cardiology/American Heart Association clinical competence statement on echocardiography: a report of the American College of Cardiology (ACC)/American Heart Association(AHA)/ American College of Physicians (ACP)/American Society of Internal Medicine (ASIM) Task Force on Clinical Competence. *Circulation.* 2003;107:1068–1089.

Chapter 2: Surface Anatomy of the Heart

1. Standring S. *Gray's Anatomy: The Anatomical Basis of Clinical Practice. Heart and Great Vessels*. Amsterdam: Elsevier Science; 2004:995–1028.

2. Lumley JSP. *Surface Anatomy. The Anatomical Basis of Clinical Examination*, 2nd ed. Edinburgh: Churchill Livingstone; 1996.

3. Malouf JF, Edwards WD, Jamil Tajik A, et al. Functional Anatomy of the Heart. In: Fuster V, O'Rourke RA, Poole-Wilson P. *Hurst's The Heart*, 12th ed. New York: McGraw Hill Medical; 2008: 45–86.

4. Bulwer BE, Rivero J, Solomon SD. Basic principles of echocardiography and tomographic anatomy. In: Solomon SD (ed.), Braunwald E (series ed.). *Atlas of Echocardiography*, 2nd ed. Philadelphia: Current Science; 2008:1–24.

Chapter 2: Echocardiographic Imaging Planes, Coronary Artery Territories, and Left Ventricular Segments (ASE)

1. Cerqueira MD, Weissman NJ, Dilsizian V, et al. Standardized Myocardial Segmentation and Nomenclature. *Circulation*. 2002;105:539–542. (Compare with Figures 6.10, 6.23, 6.65, 7.13, 7.36, 7.42.)

Chapter 3: Optimal Image Acquisition and Instrument Controls

1. Bulwer BE, Shernan SK. Optimizing the two-dimensional echocardiographic imaging. In: Savage RM, Aronson S (eds.), *Comprehensive Textbook of Intraoperative Transesophageal Echocardiography*. Philadelphia: Lippincott Williams & Wilkins; 2010.

Chapter 3: Selected Knobology and Instrumentation Basics

1. Bulwer BE, Rivero J, Solomon SD. Basic principles of echocardiography and tomographic anatomy. In: Solomon SD (ed.), Braunwald E (series ed.). *Atlas of Echocardiography*, 2nd ed. Philadelphia: Current Science; 2008:1–24.
2. Bulwer BE, Shernan SK, Thomas J. Physics of echocardiography. In: Savage RM, Aronson S (eds.). *Comprehensive Textbook of Intraoperative Transesophageal Echocardiography*. Philadelphia: Lippincott Williams & Wilkins; 2010:in press.

Chapter 4: Blood Flow Velocity Profiles

1. O'Rourke MF, Nichols WW. The nature of flow in a liquid. In: O'Rourke MF, Nichols WW (eds.). *McDonald's Blood Flow in Arteries*, 5th ed. New York: Oxford University Press; 2005:11–48.
2. O'Rourke MF, Nichols WW. Ultrasonic blood flow and velocimetry. In: O'Rourke MF, Nichols WW (eds.). *McDonald's Blood Flow in Arteries*, 5th ed. New York: Oxford University Press; 2005:149–163.
3. Hatle L, Angelsen B. Physics of blood flow. In: Hatle L, Angelsen B (eds.). *Doppler Ultrasound in Cardiology: Physical Principles and Clinical Applications*, 2nd ed. Philadelphia: Lea & Febiger; 1985:8–31.

Chapter 4: Optimizing Color Flow Doppler Controls

1. Kisslo J, Adams DB, Belkin RN. *Doppler Color-Flow Imaging*. New York: Churchill Livingstone; 1988.

2. Weyman A. Principles of color flow mapping. In: Weyman A (ed.). *Principles and Practice of Echocardiography,* 2nd ed. Philadelphia: Lea & Febiger; 1994: 218–233.

3. Lee R. Physical principles of flow mapping in cardiology. In: *Textbook of Color Doppler Echocardiography.* Philadelphia: Lea & Febiger; 1989:18–49.

Chapter 4: Pressure-Velocity Relationship: The Bernoulli Equation

1. Hatle L, Angelsen B. *Doppler Ultrasound in Cardiology: Physical Principles and Clinical Applications,* 2nd ed. Philadelphia: Lea & Febiger; 1985.

Chapter 4: Graphical Display of Doppler Frequency Spectra

1. Weyman A. Doppler signal processing. In: Weyman A (ed.). *Principles and Practice of Echocardiography,* 2nd ed. Philadelphia: Lea & Febiger; 1994:201–217.

2. Hatle L, Angelsen B. Blood velocity measurements using the Doppler effect of backscattered ultrasound. In: Hatle L, Angelsen B (eds.). *Doppler Ultrasound in Cardiology: Physical Principles and Clinical Applications,* 2nd ed. Philadelphia: Lea & Febiger; 1985:32–73.

3. Quiñones MA, Otto CM, Stoddard M, Waggoner A, Zoghbi WA. Doppler Quantification Task Force of the Nomenclature and Standards Committee of the American Society of Echocardiography. Recommendations for quantification of Doppler echocardiography: a report from the Doppler Quantification Task Force of the Nomenclature and Standards Committee of the American Society of Echocardiography. *J Am Soc Echocardiogr.* 2002;2:167–168.

4. Weyman A. Doppler instrumentation. In: Weyman A (ed.). *Principles and Practice of Echocardiography,* 2nd ed. Philadelphia: Lea & Febiger; 1994:163–183.

5. Kremkau F. *Doppler Ultrasound: Principles and Instruments,* 7th ed. Philadelphia: W.B. Saunders Company; 1990.

Chapter 4: Pulsed Doppler Velocity Profile: Left Ventricular Outflow

1. Hatle L, Angelsen B. Physics of blood flow. In: Hatle L, Angelsen B (eds.). *Doppler Ultrasound in Cardiology: Physical Principles and Clinical Applications,* 2nd ed. Philadelphia: Lea & Febiger; 1985:8–31.

2. Weyman A. Principles of flow. In: Weyman A (ed.). *Principles and Practice of Echocardiography,* 2nd ed. Philadelphia: Lea & Febiger; 1994:184–200.

Chapter 4: TDI-Derived Measures: Velocity, Displacement, Strain, and Strain Rate

1. Thomas JD, Popovic ZB. Assessment of left ventricular function by cardiac ultrasound. *J Am Coll Cardiol.* 2006;48:2012–2025.

2. Kirkpatrick JN, Vannan MA, Narula J, Lang RM. Echocardiography in heart failure: applications, utility, and new horizons. *J Am Coll Cardiol.* 2007;50: 381–396.

3. Buckberg GD, Weisfeldt ML, Ballester M, et al. Left ventricular form and function: scientific priorities and strategic planning for development of new views of disease. *Circulation.* 2004;110:e333–e336.

4. Torrent-Guasp F, Ballester M, Buckberg GD, et al. Spatial orientation of the ventricular muscle band: physiologic contribution and surgical implications. *J Thorac Cardiovasc Surg.* 2001;122:389–392.

5. Sengupta PP, Korinek J, Belohlavek M, et al. Left ventricular structure and function: basic science for cardiac imaging. *J Am Coll Cardiol.* 2006;48: 1988–2001.

Chapter 4: Ultrasound Artifacts

1. Otto C. Principles of echocardiographic image acquisition and Doppler analysis. In: Otto C (ed.). *Textbook of Clinical Echocardiography,* 2nd ed. Philadelphia: W.B. Saunders Company; 2004:1–28.

2. AMA Council on Scientific Affairs: Medical diagnostic ultrasound instrumentation and clinical interpretation: report of the Ultrasonography Task Force. *JAMA.* 1991;265:1155–1159.

3. Hedrick WR, Peterson CL. Image artifacts in real-time ultrasound. *J Diagn Med Sonog.* 1995;11:300–308.

4. Keogh F, Cooperberg PL. Is it real or is it an artifact. *Ultrasound Q.* 2001;17:201–210.

5. Kremkau W, Taylor KJ. Artifacts in ultrasound imaging. *J Ultrasound Med.* 1986;5:227–237.

6. Scanlan KA. Sonographic artifacts and their origins. *Am J Roentgenol.* 1991;156(6):1267–1272.

Chapter 5: Transducer Scan Plane, Index Mark, and Scan Sector Image Display

1. Henry WL, DeMaria A, Gramiak R, et al. Report of the American Society of Echocardiography Report on Nomenclature and Standards in Two-Dimensional Echocardiography. *Circulation.* 1980;62:212.

Chapter 5: Tips for Optimizing Image Acquisition for 2D Measurements

1. Adapted from: Recommendations for Chamber Quantification: A Report from the American Society of Echocardiography's Guidelines and Standards Committee and the Chamber Quantification Writing Group, Developed in

Conjunction with the European Association of Echocardiography, a Branch of the European Society of Cardiology. *J Am Soci Echocardiogr.* 2005;18: 1440–1463.

Chapter 5: Examination Protocol: 2D Transthoracic Echocardiography

1. Henry WL, DeMaria A, Gramiak R, et al. Report of the American Society of Echocardiography Report on Nomenclature and Standards in Two-Dimensional Echocardiography. *Circulation.* 1980;62:212.
2. Bulwer BE, Rivero J. Protocols and nomenclature in transthoracic echocardiography. In: Solomon SD (ed.), Bulwer BE (assoc. ed.). *Essential Echocardiography. A Practical Casebook with DVD.* Totowa, NJ: Humana Press; 2007:35–70.

Chapter 6: PLAX View: Scan Plane, Anatomy, and Scan Sector Display

1. Weyman AE. Standard Plane Positions—Standard Imaging Planes. In: Weyman AE (ed.). *Cross-Sectional Echocardiographic Examination.* Philadelphia: Lea & Febiger;1982:98–136.

Chapter 6: PLAX View: 3D Perspectives

1. Hung J, Lang R, Flachskampf F, et al. American Society of Echocardiography Position paper on 3D echocardiography: a review of the current status and future directions. *J Am Soc Echocardiogr.* 2007;20:213–233.

Chapter 6: PLAX View: 2D and Linear Measurements

1. Lang RM, Bierig M, Devereux B, et al. Recommendations for Chamber Quantification: A Report from the American Society of Echocardiography's Guidelines and Standards Committee and the Chamber Quantification Writing Group, Developed in Conjunction with the European Association of Echocardiography, a Branch of the European Society of Cardiology. *J Am Soci Echocardiography.* 2005;18:1440–1463.

Chapter 6: Grading Regional Wall Motion

1. Lang RM, Bierig M, Devereux B, et al. Recommendations for Chamber Quantification: A Report from the American Society of Echocardiography's Guidelines and Standards Committee and the Chamber Quantification Writing Group, Developed in Conjunction with the European Association of Echocardiography, a Branch of the European Society of Cardiology. *J Am Soci Echocardiography.* 2005;18:1440–1463.

Chapter 6: RV Inflow View: Continuous-Wave (CW) Doppler Examination of the Tricuspid Valve

1. Kirkpatrick JN, Vannan MA, Narula J, Lang RM. Echocardiography in heart failure: applications, utility, and new horizons. *J Am Coll Cardiol.* 2007;50: 381–396.

Chapter 7: A4C: Left Atrial Dynamics

1. Maccio S, Perrino P. The role of the left atrium. In: Smiseth OA, Tandera M (eds.). *Diastolic Heart Failure.* London: Springer; 2008:53–70.
2. Hitch DC, Nolan SP. Descriptive analysis of instantaneous left atrial volume—with special reference to left atrial function. *J Surg Res.* 1981;30(2):110–120.

Chapter 7: A4C: Pulmonary Venous Flow Doppler Assessment

1. Keren G, Sherez J, Megidish R, Levitt B, Laniado S. Pulmonary venous flow pattern—its relationship to cardiac dynamics. A pulsed Doppler echocardiographic study. *Circulation.* 1985;71(6):1105–1112.
2. Chen YT, Kan MN, Lee AY, Chen JS, Chiang BN. Pulmonary venous flow: its relationship to left atrial and mitral valve motion. *J Am Soc Echocardiogr.* 1993;6:387–394.
3. Rossvoll O, Hatle LK. Pulmonary venous flow velocities recorded by transthoracic Doppler ultrasound: relation to left ventricular diastolic pressures. *J Am Coll Cardiol.* 1993;7:1687–1696.

Chapter 7: A4C: Transmitral LV Inflow Doppler Assessment

1. Appleton CP, Jensen JL, Hatle LK, Oh JK. Doppler evaluation of left and right ventricular diastolic function: a technical guide for obtaining optimal flow velocity recordings. *J Am Soc Echocardiogr.* 1997;10:271–292.
2. Cohen GI, Pietrolungo JF, Thomas JD, Klein AL. A practical guide to assessment of ventricular diastolic function using Doppler echocardiography. *J Am Coll Cardiol.* 1996;27:1753–1760.
3. Aurigemma GP, Gaasch WH. Clinical practice. Diastolic heart failure. *N Engl J. Med.* 2004;351(11):1097–1105.
4. Appleton CP, Hatle LK, Popp RL. Relation of transmitral flow velocity patterns to left ventricular diastolic function: new insights from a combined hemodynamic and Doppler echocardiographic study. *J Am Coll Cardiol.* 1988;12: 426–440.
5. Lin G, Oh GK. Echocardiographic assessment of diastolic function and diagnosis of diastolic heart failure. In: Smiseth OA, Tandera M (eds.). *Diastolic Heart Failure.* London: Springer, 2008:149–162.

Chapter 7: Optimal Doppler Tissue Imaging (DTI or TDI) Technique (Figures 4.24, 7.22, 7.23)

1. Farias CA, Rodriguez L, Garcia MJ, Sun JP, Klein AL, Thomas JD. Assessment of diastolic function by tissue Doppler echocardiography: comparison with standard transmitral and pulmonary venous flow. *J Am Soc Echocardiogr.* 1999;12:609–617.
2. Nagueh SF, Middleton KJ, Kopelen HA, Zoghbi WA, Quinones MA. Doppler tissue imaging: a noninvasive technique for evaluation of left ventricular relaxation and estimation of filling pressures. *J Am Coll Cardiol.* 1997;30:1527–1533.
3. Nishimura RA, Tajik AJ. Evaluation of diastolic filling of left ventricle in health and disease: Doppler echocardiography is the clinician's Rosetta Stone. *J Am Coll Cardiol.* 1997;30:8–18.
4. Zile MR, Baicu CF, Gaasch WH. Diastolic heart failure—abnormalities in active relaxation and passive stiffness of the left ventricle. *N Engl J Med.* 2004;350:1953–1959.

Chapter 8: Findings and Summaries

1. Lang RM, Bierig M, Devereux B, et al. Recommendations for Chamber Quantification: A Report from the American Society of Echocardiography's Guidelines and Standards Committee and the Chamber Quantification Writing Group, Developed in Conjunction with the European Association of Echocardiography, a Branch of the European Society of Cardiology. *J Am Soci Echocardiography.* 18:2005:1440–1463.
2. Zornoff LA, Skali H, Pfeffer MA, St John SM, Rouleau JL, Lamas GA, et al. Right ventricular dysfunction and risk of heart failure and mortality after myocardial infarction. *J Am Coll Cardiol.* 2002;39:1450–1455.

Chapter 8: SC-Inferior Vena Cava and Right Atrial Pressure Estimates

1. Moreno FL, Hagan AD, Holmen JR, Pryor TA, Strickland RD, Castle CH. Evaluation of size and dynamics of the inferior vena cava as an index of right-sided cardiac function. *Am J Cardiol.* 1984;53:579–585.
2. Lang RM, Bierig M, Devereux B, et al. Recommendations for Chamber Quantification: A Report from the American Society of Echocardiography's Guidelines and Standards Committee and the Chamber Quantification Writing Group, Developed in Conjunction with the European Association of Echocardiography, a Branch of the European Society of Cardiology. *J Am Soci Echocardiography.* 2005;18:1440–1463.
3. Kircher BJ, Himelman RB, Schiller NB. Noninvasive estimation of right atrial pressure from the inspiratory collapse of the inferior vena cava. *Am J Cardiol.* 1990;66:493–496.

4. Zornoff LA, Skali H, Pfeffer MA, et al. Right ventricular dysfunction and risk of heart failure and mortality after myocardial infarction. *J Am Coll Cardiol.* 2002;39:1450–1455.

Chapter 8: Findings and Summaries

1. Bruce CJ, Spittell PC, Montgomery SC, Bailey KR, Tajik AJ, Seward JB. Personal ultrasound imager: abdominal aortic aneurysm screening. *J Am Soc Echocardiogr.* 2000;13:674–679.
2. Vourvouri EC, Poldermans D, Schinkel AFL, et al. Abdominal aortic aneurysm screening using a hand-held ultrasound device. A pilot study. *Eur J Vasc Endovasc Surg.* 2001;22:352–354.

Chapter 11: Utility versus Competency

1. Seward JB, Douglas PS, Erbel R, et al. Hand-carried cardiac ultrasound (HCU) device: recommendations regarding new technology. A report from the Echocardiography Task Force on New Technology of the Nomenclature and Standards Committee of the American Society of Echocardiography. *J Am Soc Echocardiogr.* 2002;15(4):369–373.

Chapter 11: Levels of Training in Echocardiography

1. AS Pearlman, JM Gardin, RP Martin, et al. Guidelines for optimal physician training in echocardiography. In: Recommendations of the American Society of Echocardiography Committee for Physician Training in Echocardiography. *Am J Cardiol.* 1987;60:158–163.

Chapter 12: The Echocardiography Examination Report

1. Gardin JM, Adams DB, Douglas PS, et al. American Society of Echocardiography. Recommendations for a standardized report for adult transthoracic echocardiography: a report from the American Society of Echocardiography's Nomenclature and Standards Committee and Task Force for a Standardized Echocardiography Report. *J Am Soc Echocardiogr.* 2002;15(3):275–290.

INDEX